Guide to the Psychiatry of Old Age

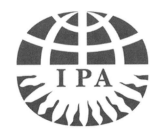

Guide to the Psychiatry of Old Age

David Ames
National Ageing Research Institute and
University of Melbourne, Australia

Edmond Chiu
University of Melbourne, Australia

James Lindesay
University of Leicester, UK

Kenneth I. Shulman
University of Toronto, Canada

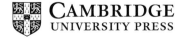

CAMBRIDGE
UNIVERSITY PRESS

CAMBRIDGE UNIVERSITY PRESS
Cambridge, New York, Melbourne, Madrid, Cape Town, Singapore,
São Paulo, Delhi, Dubai, Tokyo

Cambridge University Press
The Edinburgh Building, Cambridge CB2 8RU, UK

Published in the United States of America by Cambridge University Press, New York

www.cambridge.org
Information on this title: www.cambridge.org/9780521681919

© D. Ames, E. Chiu, J. Lindesay and K. I. Shulman 2010

This publication is in copyright. Subject to statutory exception
and to the provisions of relevant collective licensing agreements,
no reproduction of any part may take place without the written
permission of Cambridge University Press.

First published 2010

Printed in the United Kingdom at the University Press, Cambridge

A catalogue record for this publication is available from the British Library

ISBN 978-0-521-68191-9 Paperback

Cambridge University Press has no responsibility for the persistence or
accuracy of URLs for external or third-party internet websites referred to in
this publication, and does not guarantee that any content on such websites is,
or will remain, accurate or appropriate.

Every effort has been made in preparing this book to provide accurate and up-to-date information
which is in accord with accepted standards and practice at the time of publication. Although case
histories are drawn from actual cases, every effort has been made to disguise the identities of the
individuals involved. Nevertheless, the authors, editors and publishers can make no warranties that
the information contained herein is totally free from error, not least because clinical standards are
constantly changing through research and regulation. The authors, editors and publishers therefore
disclaim all liability for direct or consequential damages resulting from the use of material contained
in this book. Readers are strongly advised to pay careful attention to information provided by the
manufacturer of any drugs or equipment that they plan to use.

Contents

Foreword

By the time I launched the first dementia programme at Johns Hopkins in 1979, the psychiatry of old age was well established in the UK. Two small gems from those early days of geriatric psychiatry in the UK – the sections on old age psychiatry in *Clinical Psychiatry* by Mayer-Gross, Slater and Roth and the monograph by Felix Post, *Clinical Psychiatry of Late Life* – influenced my decision to pursue a career in the psychiatry of old age.

This new, brief guide makes geriatric psychiatry accessible to generalists, clinicians not medically trained, and even patients and families. Such efforts are needed in these days of ageing populations and shrinking resources to persuade doctors and the public to reject the prejudice of ageism, and to teach that clinical signs and symptoms of elderly patients are the products of diseases and vulnerabilities, just as they are in younger people, and not the inevitable consequences of ageing which require the discovery of the fountain of youth before the ills of the elderly can be prevented and cured.

In addition to the recognition and explanation of pathological processes causing signs and symptoms, this book promotes the narrative, or meaningful, approach, which illuminates the dignity and right to life of the elderly. The privilege of sharing the stories of almost completed lives is one of the rewards of geriatric practice. In an attempt to demonstrate this to a class of medical students, I interviewed a distinguished 90-year-old American psychiatrist, Mandel Cohen. I expected him to describe the changes he experienced as he grew older. I asked, 'Doctor, what is it like to be old?' He replied, 'I don't feel old in my mind', and he wasn't. Another story that illustrates the dignity of old people and their right to life emerged on an Alzheimer's disease (AD) unit in a nursing home. The question arose as to the validity of documents signed by family members requesting that patients not be resuscitated. In order to answer this question, I gathered a group of 10 severely impaired residents, none of whom had a Mini-mental State Examination (MMSE) score greater than 10 out of 30, and asked them if they wanted to be resuscitated..When one said, 'what does "resuscitated" mean', another member of the group said, 'you know, brought back to life'. The first person responded 'well, you have to make allowances for people with memory trouble.' Seven of 10 said they wanted resuscitation. The ones who didn't appeared to be depressed. Too often, we fail to honour the dignity of cognitively impaired elderly by asking them if they want to live, and if they don't want to live by giving them the benefit of an examination to determine if their decision was the product of a pathological process causing dementia or depression.

I would highlight a few aspects of the contemporary assessment, diagnosis and treatment of psychiatric disorders of the elderly surveyed by this book. The first is the importance of using a quantitative cognitive examination for clinical decision-making and for educating patients and families. Although cognitive examinations can be performed by specialists such as neuropsychologists, the treating clinician should examine the patient and be able to explain the results in appropriate terms to the patient and family. The important point here is not which of the several available tests is used, but that clinicians should use some quantitative method suitable for the clinical situation and purpose. Just as medicine was advanced by the introduction of the thermometer, psychiatry has been advanced by the introduction of quantitative methods of assessment. Before the modern thermometer was introduced 150 years ago, physicians felt the skin temperature and judged whether it was too warm. This method was good enough to appreciate the importance of fever, but it was not good enough to measure reliably whether the temperature was rising or falling. Today, it is not enough for the clinician to say that a patient is confused when it is possible to describe quantitatively the severity of the various impairments and to determine by serial measurement whether impairments are improving or worsening.

The second issue I would like to emphasize is the authors' discussion of that murky diagnostic category, pseudodementia. This term was usually intended to mean that a patient's cognitive impairment was not due to a neuropathological abnormality, and it implied that all true dementias were irreversible. Pseudodementia was usually applied to elderly persons with depression and cognitive impairment. Follow-up studies indicate that many of the patients so labelled do deteriorate and some have AD. This kind of evidence has been influential in returning the term dementia to its intended usage: deterioration of multiple cognitive functions in clear consciousness, without specifying either aetiology or reversibility. Instead of pseudodementia, designations such as 'depression with cognitive impairment' or 'dementia of depression' are better descriptors of the condition. This usage also encourages the point of view that depression in the elderly, both in the presence and absence of AD, should be a focus of treatment.

Finally, I would like to draw attention to the authors' discussion of currently used medications and their side effects. In some circumstances, 'reverse pharmacology' – stopping many if not all medications – leads to cognitive improvement. In other circumstances, doctors recommend medications even though treatment options are limited, because there are no curative drugs and the available symptomatic remedies carry substantial risk. In this unhappy situation, the doctors must explain the options to the patient and family and encourage them to collaborate in the decision as to whether the benefits are greater than the risks. This discussion is useful because it offers hope that something can be done or at least that no harm will be done, and it conveys to the patient and family the physicians' respect for cognitively impaired people, who often perceive that their clinicians do not consider them worthy of their efforts.

This brief guide is a welcome addition to the distinguished publications about geriatric psychiatry from the UK and more recently from many other countries. In addition to introducing the field to students and gener-alists, this brief book might even persuade some young student to join the field, just as 40 years ago one small book and a small part of a larger book written by their predecessors steered me into a satisfying career which gave me the opportunity to teach, to learn from, and to collaborate with many elderly patients and their families in order to enable them to choose to live as best they could given their individual circumstances.

Marshal Folstein MD,
Miami Beach, 2009

Preface

With rapid ageing of the world population, the psychiatry of old age (POA) has become a crucial discipline, because rates of dementia, delirium and late-life functional psychiatric disorders such as depression are increasing quickly in both the developed and developing world as a consequence of the sustained and unprecedented increase in the number of older people. In many developed countries, the subspecialty of psychiatry of old age (also known as old age psychiatry, psychogeriatrics, geriatric psychiatry and geropsychiatry) is now well established, with over 500 subspecialists in the UK and 200 in Australia. Special training programmes for the discipline have been operating in several countries for some years now, and often completion of these programmes leads to the award of a certificate of competence in the psychiatry of old age. In developing countries, especially those with rising affluence, there is emerging interest in the subspecialty and recognition of the need for service providers to acquire expertise in the area. In addition, most basic training programmes for general psychiatrists now require some exposure to and knowledge of POA, and we hope that this trend will strengthen as old people approach one-quarter of the total population in many places.

Despite this need, although there are excellent comprehensive, detailed and expensive texts on POA, there are fewer good, short, inexpensive books on this subject, and those that exist tend to have a national rather than an international focus.

For this reason, supported by Cambridge University Press (CUP) and with the endorsement of the International Psychogeriatric Association (IPA), the four of us resolved to write a book on POA that would be short, comprehensive and affordable. In making this decision, we were mindful both of an apparent unmet need and the involvement that all four of us have had with IPA over many years (all of us have been members of IPA's Board of Directors, EC was IPA secretary and then president, and DA has edited IPA's peer-reviewed journal *International Psychogeriatrics* since 2003). This, after a prolonged gestation and writing process, is the result. It is aimed at trainee psychiatrists, higher trainees in the psychiatry of old age, geriatricians and trainee geriatricians, general psychiatrists, neurologists, physicians in training, general practitioners, allied health staff, nurses and medical students. We hope that our audience will be international, so the book's content is not limited solely to the experience of POA in the three countries in which the authors have lived and worked, but is informed by our experience of visiting, teaching and talking to our colleagues in a wide variety of countries around the world.

In order to keep the book to a relatively manageable size, the text is not referenced with citations for every statement made, but we hope that the suggestions for further reading given at the end of each chapter (many of which are available free of charge to members of IPA) will be found to be up to date and helpful.

We trust that health practitioners around the world will find this to be a useful book and that in due course a second edition will be needed. To that end we encourage readers to suggest to us how this edition could be improved (contact David Ames on dames@unimelb.edu.au).

Books like this do not appear without the help and assistance of a large number of people. We are grateful to Richard Marley and his colleagues at CUP (CUP is an IPA corporate partner and has published *International Psychogeriatrics*, IPA's peer-reviewed journal, since 2004) for their encouragement to write the book and their patience when the first author's numerous other responsibilities slowed down its creation. Nisha Doshi worked hard to help us get the book into production, then Jo Endell-Cooper and Sara Brunton refined the copy that was submitted into the elegant text that you now hold. Susan Oster, the executive director of IPA, was consistently enthusiastic about this project, especially the idea of offering copies to IPA members at discounted cost. Leonardo Pantoni (IPA publications committee chair) and Michael Philpot (book review editor of *International Psychogeriatrics*) checked the text rapidly at short notice to ensure that its content was compatible with IPA's mission and values, and we are very grateful to them for doing this so quickly and cheerfully, and for their many useful and thoughtful suggestions which improved the final text. Roz Seath gave tireless and invaluable secretarial support to this project, as she has done for more books than we, or she, would care to count. The book was completed during the last three months of 2009 when DA was on sabbatical leave from his research institute and university – the hospitality and kindness of Craig Ritchie and his Imperial College colleagues at Charing Cross Hospital, London during this time helped to make possible the book's completion. Finally, we would like to thank our patients and their families – from them we have learned most of what little we know about this expanding and intriguing branch of medicine.

David Ames, Edmond Chiu, James Lindesay, Ken Shulman
London, Melbourne, Leicester, Toronto
December 2009

Abbreviations

AAMI	age-associated memory impairment
ACE	angiotensin converting enzyme
Ach	acetylcholine
AD	Alzheimer's disease
ADAS-Cog	Alzheimer's Diesease Assessment Scale Cognitive subscale
ADI	Alzheimer's Disease International
ADL	activities of daily living
ApoE	apolipoprotein E
APP	amyloid precursor protein
BPSD	Behavioural and Psychological Symptoms of Dementia
CAM	Confusion Assessment Method
CAMCOG	Cambridge Cognitive Examination
CDT	Clock Drawing Test
CERAD	Consortium to Establish a Registry for Alzheimer's Disease
CIND	cognitive impairment not dementia
CMAI	Cohen Mansfield Agitation Inventory
CVAE	cerebrovascular adverse event
DLB	dementia with Lewy bodies,
DRS	Delirium Rating Scale
ECA	Epidemiologic Catchment Area
ECT	electroconvulsive therapy
EOS	early-onset schizophrenia
FAB	frontal assessment battery
FBE	full blood examination
FTD	frontotemporal dementias
GAD	generalized anxiety
HGA	hypothalamus–pituitary–gonadal
HPA	hypothalamus–pituitary–adrenal
HPI	history of present illness
IPA	International Psychogeriatric Association
LOS	late-onset schizophrenia
MAOI	monoamine oxidase inhibitor
MCI	mild cognitive impairment
MEG	magneto-encephalography
MMSE	Mini-mental State Examination
MoCA	Montreal Cognitive Assessment

NMDA	N-methyl-D-aspartate
NSAID	non-steroidal anti-inflammatory drug
PDD	Parkinson's Disease Dementia
PET	Positron Emission Tomography
POA	psychiatry of old age
RBF	Regional Blood Flow
RCT	randomized controlled trial
RUDAS	Rowland Universal Dementia Assessment Scale
SPET	Single Photon Emission Tomography
TCA	tricyclic antidepressant
TIA	transient ischaemic attack
VaD	vascular dementia
VBR	Ventricular Brain Ratio
VLOSP	Very-late-onset schizophrenia-like psychosis
WMH	white matter hyperintensity

What is the psychiatry of old age and why do we need it?

The psychiatry of old age (POA) is concerned with the identification, assessment, treatment and care of older adults with mental disorders, and of those who look after them. Mental illness in late life is as old as humanity, and there is a long history of social and medical interventions with affected individuals – some more enlightened than others. In all societies and at all times the care of elderly people has been grounded in the family, and it is only when this source of support is absent or insufficient that the local community or the State has intervened. In mediaeval Europe, the legislation developed for this purpose had as much to do with the management of property as the welfare of the individual, but the records show that in the context of small and relatively cohesive communities it could deliver sophisticated and effective care for insane and incompetent individuals, both rich and poor. The modern history of old age psychiatry in developed societies has its origins in the changing social demography of the nineteenth century, with the rapid urbanization of populations and growth in the numbers of elderly people. With local community support no longer sustainable, the poor and the disabled (elderly people were often both) were particularly vulnerable. The responses to this welfare challenge were many and various, and included Poor Laws, pensions, and institutional solutions such as workhouses, infirmaries, and the lunatic asylums. It was within these institutions, often later re-labelled as 'hospitals', that the frailties of old age were medicalized, and became the professional responsibility of physicians and psychiatrists. So far as mental illness was concerned, however, this was not a responsibility that was especially welcomed by anyone. In particular, elderly people with dementia were felt to be a nuisance; they could not be discharged from acute medical beds, psychiatrists were not interested in them, and no-one had anything to offer beyond institutional warehousing in nursing homes or the back-wards of the old asylums.

This professional pessimism and lack of interest began to be challenged in the second half of the twentieth century by small groups of innovators, particularly in the UK. The creation of 'geriatric medicine' within the new National Health Service (NHS), with its avowed interest in all of the physical and mental problems of older people, and its multi-professional approach to solving them, was an important model for the later development of old age psychiatry by its pioneers, figures such as Tom Arie and Tony Whitehead. An important factor influencing this change of attitude in service providers was research, for example that by Martin (later Sir Martin) Roth in the UK, demonstrating that not all mental illness in old age has the same bad prognosis, and that mortality in individuals with affective and psychotic disorders was much less than in those with demen-tia. This optimism was encouraged by the successful application of both physical and social treatments to elderly patients. A number of large-scale epidemiologi-cal studies of mental disorders in elderly community populations were carried out at this time in the USA, Scandinavia, and the UK, which characterized the full range of these conditions, and the extent to which those affected by them were out of touch with any services. These surveys also made it clear that only a minority of the elderly population were mentally ill; an important message from the emerging science of gerontology was that physical and mental frailty was by no means the inevitable consequence of ageing, and that the compression of morbidity was a realistic and achievable goal.

Another important factor that has driven change in service provision for eld-erly people in developed societies has been government health policy, developed in response to demographic ageing, the cost-effectiveness of treatment and care, and rising expectations of the population regarding the quality of that care. By the 1960s, it was widely accepted that the traditional custodial approach to the care of the mentally ill was no longer acceptable, and that the focus of services should move to the home and the community. However, the rate and extent of the development of community-based old-age psychiatry services have differed substantially in different countries; those with universal health and social care funding and centralized health policy and planning, such as the UK and Canada, have created much more comprehensive services than those without, such as the USA. Active and vocal voluntary and other non-government organizations, such as the Alzheimer's Association (USA), Alzheimer's Society (UK) and Alzheimer's Disease International (ADI), have also been a valuable stimulus to service devel-opment, particularly for the support of carers. The development of services for the elderly mentally ill, and the international consensus model of their organ-ization published by the World Psychiatric Association in 1997, are discussed in detail in Chapter 11.

The future

Developed societies may have been the first to experience demographic ageing and the growth in the number of elderly people with mental illness, but the rest of the world is catching up fast. According to a recent review, there are currently 24.3 million people with dementia in the world, with 4.6 million new cases annu-ally. The number of those affected by dementia is projected to double every 20 years, with 42.3 million people worldwide living with dementia in 2020, and 81.1 million in 2040. Most of these people with dementia live in the developing world: 60% in 2001, rising to 71% in 2040. This review identified three groups of countries: the developed regions, which start from a high base rate of demen-tia and which will experience moderate proportional increases in numbers of affected individuals of about 100% between 2001 and 2040; Latin America and Africa, which start from a low base rate, and which will experience more rapid two- to threefold increases in prevalence by 2040; and India, China, South Asia and the Western Pacific regions, which both start from a high base rate and will experience at least threefold increases in prevalence. By 2040, there will be three times as many people with dementia in this third group of countries than there will be in Western Europe.

Of course, dementia is not the only disorder that will increase in prevalence with demographic ageing. Other conditions such as vascular disease, arthritis, and sensory impairments will all contribute to an increasing burden of chronic physical and mental disability in old age, as will emerging problems such as the global epidemic of obesity. Other factors are also likely to have an impact upon the future welfare and care of elderly people. For example, in developed societies, the shifting dependency ratio of the population will require individuals to continue working beyond traditional retirement age, just as they always have done in poorer countries. Increased geographic mobility, with children moving away from home and parents relocating on retirement, will reduce the availability of informal care, as will the continued growth in the number of single-person households. In the developing world, there will be the problem of the competing demands of young and old for health care, particularly for conditions such as AIDS that disproportionately affect younger, economically active age groups. For some countries, rapid economic growth may help to some extent with the challenges of demographic ageing, but this will bring problems of its own, such as the economic migration of younger people into cities and to more affluent countries. In many parts of the world, the stigma associated with mental disorder at all ages is still a major obstacle to the provision of care. There are other, less predictable, eventualities that could have a major impact upon the capacity of all societies to respond to demographic ageing in the years to come, for example pandemic influenza, which may disproportionately affect the young, or climate change bringing about large-scale population movements and resource wars. On a more positive note, there would be considerable economic and social benefits globally, were we to achieve effective control of widespread endemic diseases such as malaria.

These projections and predictions have profound social and economic implications for both developed and developing societies around the world. Even the richest nations will struggle to maintain levels of health and social care at their current levels, and for much of the developing world the models of service infrastructure pioneered in the UK and other developed countries simply will not be an option. In the absence of cheap and simple cures for disorders such as dementia, other approaches will have to be found. There will need to be a much greater public health focus on primary prevention, particularly the prevention of cerebrovascular disease through effective control of vascular risk factors such as hypertension, diabetes and smoking. The quest to develop a vaccine against Alzheimer's disease (AD) has been stalled in the early stages because of adverse effects in the initial trials, but this approach may still hold some promise, and other evidence-based novel approaches to treating AD are being developed and tried out. In the longer term, there is a growing body of evidence to indicate that the onset of clinical dementia may be delayed in individuals with a greater amount of 'cerebral reserve', suggesting that better nutrition and education in childhood and young adulthood may have a positive effect on the incidence of dementia in old age. It is not yet clear what, if anything, can be done to boost cerebral reserve in later life; the 'use it or lose it' hypothesis is attractive, but the evidence to support it is still limited. So far as secondary prevention is concerned, there will be a need to develop new service models for societies that can only afford basic levels of health care. Inevitably, these will need to build upon what already exists, for example by developing and extending the role of those professionals such as child nurses who currently visit families in their homes. The focus of their new role would be upon improved detection and family/carer support, through information, training, and developing local community solutions where possible. Public education at all levels will also be important in raising everyone's awareness and understanding of mental illness in old age, and in combating the associated stigma.

FURTHER READING

Article

Ferri, C. P. et al. (2005). Global prevalence of dementia: a Delphi consensus study. *Lancet*, 366, 2112–2117.
This paper uses published evidence to estimate the current and future global prevalence of dementia.

Book

Jacoby, R., Oppenheimer, C., Dening, T., and Thomas, A. (Eds.) (2008). *Oxford Textbook of Old Age Psychiatry.* Oxford: Oxford University Press.
Easily the best of the comprehensive guides to the subspecialty.

2

Assessing the elderly psychiatric patient

Introduction

The assessment of older adults with affective, behavioural or cognitive symptoms requires versatility and a wide range of knowledge and skills. Hence, Brice Pitt, one of the pioneers in the subspecialty, referred to the psychiatry of old age (POA) as 'general psychiatry only more so!' This chapter will outline the special features that characterize the assessment of older adults with psychiatric problems, i.e. we will focus on the 'added value' necessary to understand the elderly patient compared to a younger adult. These special features include: (1) flexibility in adapting to the most appropriate place and mode of assessment; (2) inclusion of the informant/caregiver as a fundamental and essential component of the assessment; (3) skill in taking a history that spans a lifetime; (4) special understanding of medical co-morbidity (especially neurologic disorders and the impact of drugs on the central nervous system); and (5) particular skill in cognitive screening, including frontal/executive brain functions.

Where to assess the patient

The doctor's office is not a practical setting for the assessment of any patients except for those who are high functioning, cooperative and competent. For those with significant cognitive impairment, the very frail, the resistant, and the incapable, the patient's own setting is preferred. This is not just optimal, but often necessary. This is the only way that one can properly assess the impact of environmental factors, safety issues and obtain a better sense of how the patient functions in terms of their independent activities of daily living.

Health care systems should provide incentives for physicians to leave their offices or hospitals and go to the patient's own setting. In older adults, the complex and multi-faceted nature of their clinical condition invites the involvement of other health care professionals who can address psychosocial issues and practical concerns. Ideally, the psychiatrist is part of a multi disciplinary team that has the range of expertise that can address medical, cognitive, behavioural and psychological issues while attending to practical concerns such as safety, nutrition, mobility and the well-being of caregivers (see below). A multi disciplinary team based in or closely affiliated with a general hospital setting also can have access to medical consultations and investigations. Because of the high prevalence of medical co-morbidity, access to these resources is essential. One may need to rule out common systemic medical conditions such as coronary artery disease, heart failure, hypothyroidism, vitamin deficiencies, hepatic and renal dysfunction, or electrolyte imbalances. Hence, ready access to laboratory services is necessary. Moreover, in assessing dementia and other cognitive disorders, neuroimaging is a frequent component of the assessment and differential diagnosis. Selective access to brain scanning technology (usually this will be computerized X-ray tomography (CT), magnetic resonance imaging (MRI); sometimes single photon emission tomography (SPET) will be required) is necessary to assess cerebrovascular pathology, degenerative disorders, or rule out the possibility of space-occupying lesions. For psychiatric services, this is often done in the context of attempting to differentiate mood disorders from dementias and other neurological disorders.

Because of the high frequency of medical co-morbidity and associated drug treatments, we advise that all psychiatric assessments of older adults should be preceded by an assessment by a general practitioner (GP – also known in some parts of the world as a primary care physician). All new changes in affect, behaviour or cognition should be assessed first by GPs and referred to a psychiatric service when the condition is severe, complex or poorly understood. From a primary care perspective, the issue of cognitive screening is an important public health concern which has not yet been adequately resolved. Clearly, the nature of a busy primary care practice necessitates the capacity to perform screening quickly, efficiently and effectively. This will be addressed later in this chapter.

Role of the carer/informant

The historical psychiatric culture has often excluded families from being active participants in the assessment and ongoing management of major psychiatric disorders. This has evolved partly because of legitimate concerns about confidentiality, and the primacy of the doctor/patient relationship. However, one needs to balance this need with the reality that many major mental disorders have a profound impact on families and caregivers and they justifiably have a right to be included in the treatment process. This is also because of the fundamental fact that they can provide vital information that would often be missing if they were not part of the assessment. Referring back to the Brice Pitt dictum that geriatric psychiatry is general psychiatry but 'more so', one can see that in the assessment of an older adult, the absence of a caregiver/informant severely limits the quality of the assessment and hence the ability to make the best judgements in terms of diagnosis and ongoing management. Therefore, we suggest that all psychiatric assessments of older adults should include an informant or carer who lives with the patient or has a very good understanding of the patient's functioning and behaviour. Carers and families should be considered equal partners in the therapeutic alliance that develops with the psychiatrist and the multi disciplinary health care team. The traditional dyad of 'doctor/patient relationship' needs to be transformed into the 'doctor/family relationship' in the psychiatry of old age.

A fortiori, this is the case when the patient is incapable, cognitively impaired or extremely frail and vulnerable. In this case, the caregiver is often acting in the capacity of power of attorney for personal care.

Whom to see first and whether to see patients and families individually or together is an important consideration that has not been given adequate consideration in many psychiatric textbooks. One could hold to the general principle that the patient should be seen first in order to give a sense that his/her concerns are being taken seriously. This is especially true if there is any element of suspiciousness or paranoia that is evident in the initial referral. However, one needs to be very flexible in all aspects of assessment and management. If cognitive impairment is the primary concern, there seems to be little point in spending much time and effort taking a history from a compromised individual. If it is obvious that one is dealing with a significant cognitive concern, then it is probably more efficient to interview the family member or carer first in order to obtain a better sense of the clinical picture before bringing in the patient where the primary focus will be on the mental status examination and cognitive assessment.

If the patient and family members are seen together, this may significantly inhibit the informants from providing an honest and full clinical picture. When seen together, family members or carers often attempt to help the patient who is struggling with cognitive challenges. Moreover, inter-personal dynamics often manifest during the course of the interview. Certainly, that is a reason to see the patient and family together in order to assess such interactions. However, to obtain an optimal history and cognitive examination, this is best done by separating the patient and informants for assessment purposes.

Having completed the assessment and having established a formulation and management plan, then it is best to see the patient and family together in order to minimize divergent interpretations of the assessment and management plan. Even so, this is often a challenge, but there is considerable merit in bringing everyone together at the end to summarize and give feedback.

'Clinical pearl'

As a general rule, carers are always accurate when they indicate that there has been a change in the patient's level of functioning or psychiatric status. Like mothers who report on their children's clinical status, one needs to take this report at face value. However, it has been our experience that the caregiver's interpretation of the changes in mental state or behaviour need to be viewed in a different vein. Very often, the carer's interpretation is mistaken. In particular with early dementias, carers frequently misinterpret motivational deficit and cognitive changes as a sign of depression, or attribute the changes to longstanding personality traits. Carers may feel that their loved one is being deliberately obstinate or retaliating because of inter-personal tensions or conflicts. These attributions do need to be corrected and the best time to do that is at the initial assessment.

History taking

As in general psychiatry, history taking is perhaps the most important element in establishing a provisional diagnosis. The challenge, of course, in taking a history from an 80- or 90-year-old is that one can be overwhelmed by the many details of a long life. The clinician should have the capacity to filter relevant from irrelevant material and focus on major events and patterns of behaviour in order to assess an older adult in a timely fashion. History taking does not involve a detailed description of the early development of an 85-year-old with respect to infant developmental milestones. Rather, one needs to have a general sense of whether development was normal and whether there is any history of major disruptions to normal development because of early losses of a parent from death or divorce or any significant trauma in childhood. One is interested in obtaining a general overview of the patterns of adjustment to school, social relationships, intimacy, work history, retirement, bereavement, and to the disabilities of later life. These facts need to be synthesized into a concise and coherent history rather than a detailed and over-inclusive one. Significantly, sexual history is often omitted because of embarrassment on the part of the examiner. However, changes in sexual function and activity can provide helpful clues regarding the development of mood or degenerative brain disorders, and this aspect of history taking should not be overlooked.

Age of onset is an important variable in all of psychiatry and this is just as true in later life. This will often be a clue as to the role of familial or genetic factors. Even in older adults, a detailed family history of psychiatric disorder is essential. Certainly, conditions that begin earlier in life tend to be more genetically determined and suggest a constitutional vulnerability that is greater than a late-onset mental disorder where medical/neurological disorders and the central nervous system (CNS) impact of drugs play a more central role. This has implications in terms of investigation, further assessment, diagnosis and management.

A special understanding of medical co-morbidity is an important aspect of the assessment of the older adult. This requires particular attention in the history taking, including a review of major illnesses and operations as well as a specific inquiry about any prior head injury. Furthermore, a detailed review of the current drug regimen and recent drug changes is especially important in the assessment of an older adult. Thus, the physician-assessor plays a particularly central role in the assessment of older adults for this reason. This also highlights the importance of having ready access to medical consultation and investigations.

Mental status examination

The mental status examination takes the form of a semi-structured interview and should happen throughout the history-taking process. As in mixed-age adults, the mental status examination begins from the moment one observes the patient for the first time and continues throughout the course of the assessment. What distinguishes the assessment of an older adult really focuses on the need to do a careful cognitive examination in all cases. One needs to resist the inclination to avoid a formal cognitive screen when the older adult appears to be superficially intact. Clinicians will regret this when it becomes clear later in the clinical course that a cognitive disorder was indeed emerging at the time of the initial assessment. This is especially important in individuals who maintain their social competence through the early stages of a dementing illness. This is also relevant in individuals who have been functioning at a very high premorbid level and the examiner may be hesitant to embarrass the patient. However, this is almost always a mistake and experience suggests that some form of cognitive assessment is essential in every psychiatric assessment of an older adult. How to go about doing a cognitive assessment is a technique that must be learned and then practicsed (see below).

'Clinical pearl' – 'The age and date of birth' cognitive screen

We recommend a 'clinical tip' whereby a cognitive screen occurs imperceptibly at the very outset of the interview. When taking basic demographic information such as name, address, marital, occupational or retirement status, one can determine whether there is a significant cognitive concern. This is done by asking two questions: (1) How old are you? and (2) What is your date of birth? In the context of a demographic inquiry, these are non-threatening questions but will often reveal cognitive impairment if the patient has significant difficulty recalling their age or when the age and date of birth are not congruent. This will allow the examiner to move into a more formal cognitive screen earlier in the process than would otherwise be the case.

As with younger adults, it is best to initiate the interview with open-ended questions after the basic demographic information has been determined. These open-ended questions provide two important outcomes. The first is to allow the patient to review significant ideational, psychological and emotional material without being deflected by structured and focused questions. Secondly, the open-ended questions will help to reveal evidence of thought disorder or over-inclusiveness.

Sometimes, the interviewer's reaction to a patient's history is a sense of 'vagueness'. This is often a clue that there is an underlying cognitive problem and should invite a formal, structured cognitive assessment during the interview. We certainly suggest that if the patient is inclined to be talkative, it is a worthwhile investment of one or two minutes at the outset of the interview to allow the patient free rein while carefully observing for thought content and thought process.

Assessment of appearance and behaviour, speech, thought form and content, mood, the presence of abnormal ideas or experiences and insight and judgement should proceed as would be done for any psychiatric patient. However, the cognitive assessment needs to be much more detailed than would be the case for most younger patients because of the high prevalence of cognitive disorders in this age group (see below). Patience may be required, because old people become tired more easily than young ones and are much more likely to have sensory impairments that render the assessment more complex and difficult. Sometimes, if the patient becomes fatigued easily, it will be necessary to conduct a full assessment over more than one session. Particular attention should be paid to the presence or absence of any mood symptoms (old people are sometimes reticent to admit to low mood) and it should be noted that any delusional symptoms are likely to be relatively banal and to relate to the patient's immediate surrounds and social circle, in contrast to young patients with schizophrenia in whom bizarre delusions and hallucinations are quite common.

'Clinical pearl' – 'The white roots sign'

Observation as part of mental status can be a clue to underlying diagnosis. Felix Post, one of the original pioneers in the psychiatry of old age, often referred to the 'white roots sign'. This reflects the fact that personal grooming is often a reflection of the underlying clinical status of the patient. Decline in personal grooming is often a clue to the presence of an underlying disorder. For women who are in the habit of dyeing their hair, this is a special clinical opportunity. One can posit a diagnosis of major depression by simply observing the white roots of a woman who has been in the habit of attending regularly at the hairdresser. Since major depression affects initiative and motivation, in severe cases this will impact on an older woman's long established pattern of hair care. With the knowledge that hair grows at the rate of approximately half an inch a month, a two-inch band of white roots suggests a four-month major depression. This clinical observation of course needs to be corroborated by history and the remainder of the mental status examination. However, an observation such as this can certainly establish a hypothesis earlier in the assessment. This needs to be pursued by the examiner by posing more critical questions in order to differentiate major depression from dementia, as will be described in the next chapter.

Cognitive assessment and benefits of early diagnosis

Cognitive assessment is a vital part of the overall assessment of all older adults. No matter how intact an older adult appears or how preserved the social graces, a formal cognitive screening is vital. Otherwise, the risk of missing the early stages of a cognitive disorder is very high. However, one must bear in mind the fact that no cognitive screening measure is an 'Alzheimer test'. The cognitive assessment must always be interpreted in the context of the history and other investigations in order to establish a provisional diagnosis. However, cognitive assessment can help to determine whether the impairment is diffuse or focal in nature and whether it involves primarily memory functions or frontal/executive functions as described below. Another very important aspect of cognitive screening is the ability to measure severity of impairment. No matter what cognitive instrument or battery is utilized, it can be used to monitor change over time if repeated in precisely the same fashion.

Cognitive assessment certainly will help to determine whether a dementia is present. Moreover, early detection of dementia confers a number of important potential benefits from both a clinical and societal perspective. These benefits include the value of providing an explanation to patients and families about changes in affect, behaviour or cognition that may be secondary to a dementing illness. Secondly, the early diagnosis of dementia allows for important planning opportunities, including powers of attorney, advance directives, and last Will and Testament. Furthermore, having established the diagnosis of dementia, one can be alert to the concomitant risks associated with dementia, including delirium and driving risks that must be carefully assessed and monitored. From a treatment perspective, early diagnosis may allow for potential benefits from the new cognitive enhancers whose benefit is most likely to occur in the early stages of the disease.

'Clinical pearl' – How to begin the formal cognitive assessment

When the patient spontaneously refers to memory concerns or intellectual concerns of any kind, one may seize on that opportunity to begin the more formal assessment. One should generally ask for the permission of the patient to test 'concentration and memory'. By adding the word 'concentration', this tends to defuse the anxiety that surrounds the task of 'memory testing'.

Which cognitive assessment instrument(s) to use?

A recent International Psychogeriatric Association (IPA) survey of brief cognitive screening instruments revealed that geriatric specialists worldwide are using a relatively small number of brief screening instruments. In decreasing order of frequency they include: all forms of the Mini-mental State Examination (MMSE) (100%); the Clock Drawing Test (72%); Delayed Recall (56%); Verbal Fluency (39%); Similarities (27%); and the Trail Making Test (25%). Newer brief batteries, such as the Mini-Cog combine a short memory test with the Clock Drawing Test using a simple scoring system. Other recently developed brief batteries worth considering are the Montreal Cognitive Assessment (MoCA) focused on mild cognitive impairment, the GPCOG designed for use in primary care, and the Rowland Universal Dementia Assessment Scale (RUDAS) which emphasises multi-cultural factors and is designed for use in individuals who are not fluent in the language of the examiner. The Self Test is designed to be administered with minimal supervision, while the 10-item Abbreviated Mental Test Score is still used by some specialists (see the further reading section at the end of this chapter for references to these cognitive screening instruments).

The Mini-mental State Examination ('the Folstein')

By far the most widely used cognitive screening instrument in the world is the Mini-mental State Examination developed by Folstein *et al.* in 1975. It was developed at a critical time in the history of geriatrics and hence the MMSE became 'imprinted' in the minds of clinicians ever since. Despite all of its limitations, including bias by education, culture and language, it is still the lingua franca of cognitive screening. Clinicians communicate in shorthand by quoting the MMSE score out of 30. Although variations on the MMSE have been developed, including the Standardized Mini-mental State Examination and the Modified Mini-mental State Examination, the original MMSE is still by far the most commonly utilised. The MMSE is more heavily weighted towards tests of orientation, short-term memory and language with only one visuospatial test (intersecting pentagons). The MMSE is divided into sections including orientation, registration, attention and calculation, recall and language. The MMSE does not formally test frontal lobe or execution functions and these tests need to be added as part of the cognitive assessment. Despite all the limitations of the MMSE that have been well documented, it has persisted in the clinical arena for over 30 years. As long as clinicians do not give it excessive weight from a diagnostic perspective, it remains a useful instrument in the evaluation of cognitive disorders and a signal of the need for further inquiry, investigations or monitoring.

Another limitation of the MMSE is the length of time needed to administer it. Ideally, a cognitive screening test/battery should be very short in duration, taking less than five minutes to administer. In general practice, this probably needs to be shortened to less than two minutes. In addition to brevity, the ideal qualities of a screening test should include: relative independence from culture, language and education; good psychometric properties including inter-rater reliability, test re-test reliability, a good balance of sensitivity and specificity, and a high level of predictive validity. As this book went to press, the MMSE-2, a completely revised version of the MMSE, was published. Further details are available from www.mmse.com and www.parinc.com.

The Clock Drawing Test

One very popular screening test is the Clock Drawing Test (CDT), now widely used as evidenced by the IPA survey. However, it still presents challenges with respect to an appropriate scoring system. This test generally uses a pre-drawn circle (approximately 10 cm in diameter) which is placed before the patient with the following instruction: 'This is a clock face. Please fill in the numbers and then set the time to ten past eleven'. One should avoid the use of the word 'hands' as this clue may mask impairment of higher level functions such as abstract thinking. The CDT has proven to be useful because of the wide range of intellectual functions it subsumes. It casts a wide net that includes

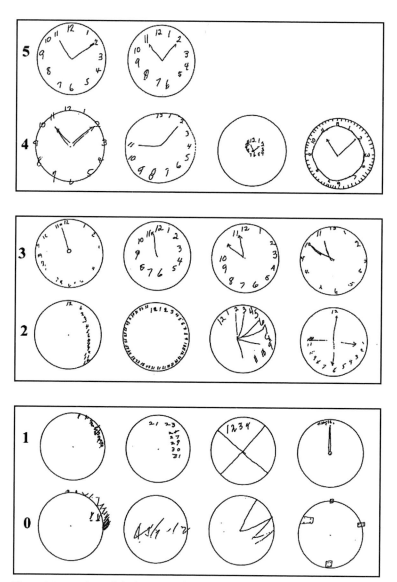

Figure 2.1 A variety of clock test results ranging from intact to severely impaired. Reproduced with permission from Shulman K. I. (2000). Clock-drawing: is it the ideal cognitive screening test? *International Journal of Geriatric* Psychiatry, **15**, 548–561.

functions such as comprehension, planning, visual memory, visuospatial ability, abstract thinking, concentration and motivation. The task of setting the time to ten past eleven involves the inhibition of the stimulus to point the hand to the number ten. Figure 2.1 shows a variety of clock test results ranging from intact to severely impaired.

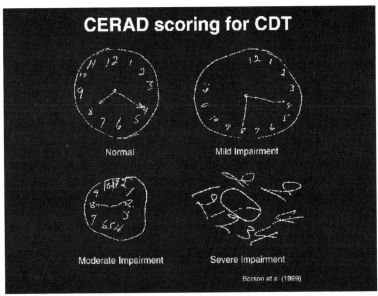

Figure 2.2 A four-point scoring system records zero for an intact clock, one point for mild impairment, two points for moderate impairment and three points for severe impairment. Reproduced from Borson *et al.* (2000), with permission from the The Gerontological Society of America. © The Gerontological Society of America.

Consensus on clock scoring has been problematic, but recent research suggests that the simpler the scoring system the better. A four-point scoring system records zero for an intact clock, one point for mild impairment, two points for moderate impairment and three points for severe impairment. This scoring system was recommended originally by the Consortium to Establish a Registry for Alzheimer's Disease (CERAD) (Figure 2.2). Recently, it has been utilized by Borson and colleagues in the development of the Mini-Cog. The Mini-Cog uses a two-step process including a test of delayed recall and the clock drawing test (Figure 2.3).

Qualitative assessment of clock drawing may be as useful as quantitative scoring. One can observe perseveration, poor planning and conceptual deficits from the clock drawing test. Like other screening instruments, the CDT lends itself to use as a monitor of change over time especially because it is a simple visual record that can be readily compared from one visit to another.

Frontal lobe/executive impairment

The frontal lobes oversee a number of important functions that include concentration and attention, verbal fluency, and abstract ability, as well as insight and judgment. The clock drawing test allows for the elicitation of frontal lobe/executive impairment through its wide cognitive screening net. However, other more specific tests are also appropriate and easily incorporated into a cognitive screen. In particular, verbal fluency has proven to be

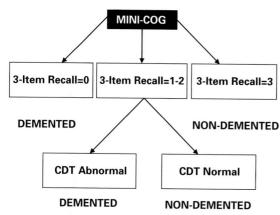

Figure 2.3 The Mini-Cog uses a two-step process including a test of delayed recall and the clock drawing test. Reproduced from Borson, S. *et al.* (2000). The Mini-Cog: a cognitive 'vital signs' measure for dementia screening in multi-lingual elderly. *International Journal of Geriatric Psychiatry*, **15**, 1021–1027, with permission from John Wiley & Sons Ltd. © John Wiley & Sons Limited.

a valid and reliable method. We use a 'phonemic' prime such as the letter 'F' with the instruction: 'List as many words as you can that begin with the letter 'F' in the next minute'. (A native speaker with high school education should be able to generate approximately 14 words.)

'Clinical pearl'

Patients with frontal lobe/executive impairment causing disinhibition may blurt out a common 'F' word as the first reaction to such a direction. We hasten to add that this is not diagnostic, as many examples of false positives are found within the general population.

Verbal fluency also includes the use of a 'semantic' prime: 'Name as many four-legged animals as you can in the next minute'. As a general rule, patients with Alzheimer's disease with mainly parietal/temporal impairment will have more difficulty with the semantic prime, while patients with primarily frontal lobe/executive dysfunction may have more difficulty with the phonemic prime. (Similar to 'F' words, an average of 14 words is expected.)

Tasks that require shifts of mental set may reveal perseveration, a non-specific but sensitive sign of brain dysfunction. This can be tested by drawing three loops and asking the patient to copy such loops and then continue the pattern across the page. Patients with perseverative responses add extra loops to the three that are recorded. One can also use a line of alternating triangles and rectangles. In the 'go-no-go' sequence, the examiner taps twice and asks the patient to tap once and then asks the patient to tap twice when the examiner taps once. Using random tapping of one or two taps allows determinationof whether the patient can adjust and switch sets accordingly, or if the patient lapses into a perseverative response by mimicking the number of taps the examiner makes.

Abstract ability is best tested by similarities such as: 'How are an orange and apple alike?'; 'What is similar about a bus and an aeroplane?'; 'What is similar about a sculpture and a painting?'

A variant of the CDT known as the CLOX test is designed to detect frontal lobe/executive impairment. In the first step (CLOX 1), the patient is asked to draw a freehand clock. If the patient is unable to do this or cannot do it accurately, the patient is then asked to copy a drawing of a completed clock (CLOX 2). If the first component (CLOX 1) is impaired but CLOX 2 is intact (copying ability is retained), this suggests frontal lobe/executive impairment (Figure 2.4).

The frontal assessment battery (FAB) includes six items and measures a range of frontal functions including mental flexibility, conceptualization, inhibitory control, motor programming and environmental autonomy. The six specific tests include: (1) similarities; (2) verbal fluency; (3) Luria three-step procedure (fist, edge, palm), a test of 'motor programming'; (4) the use of conflicting instructions 'tap twice when I tap once' alternating with 'tap once when I tap twice'; (5) go-no-go test (inhibitory control) 'tap once when I tap once' alternating with 'do not tap when I tap twice'; and (6) prehension behaviour (environmental autonomy). In this test, the patient sits with palms faced upwards resting on his/her knees. The patient is instructed not to take the examiner's hands when the examiner touches the palm of the patient. If the early instruction is ignored, repeat the instruction with the test 'now do not take my hands'.

More comprehensive cognitive assessment instruments

In addition to the tests listed here, other more comprehensive assessment instruments such as the Cambridge Cognitive Examination (CAMCOG) and the Alzheimer's Diesease Assessment Scale Cognitive subscale (ADAS-Cog) may be of use when no neuropsychologist is available and yet a more comprehensive assessment is required.

Capacity assessments

Often, clinicians are asked to respond to medico-legal requests for assessments of older adults involving various types of capacity. The range of capacities that are requested include the capacity to give instructions for power of attorney, property or personal care. There are clinical assessments involving capacity to consent to treatment as well as the capacity to consent to long-term care for frail, older adults. More complex capacities involve financial and driving capacity as well as testamentary capacity, the capacity to make out a Will.

The general cognitive assessment, as described above, is relevant in all capacity assessments as it provides a reflection of global cognitive functioning. However, it is important to note that all capacities are considered 'task-specific' and include

CLOX Test

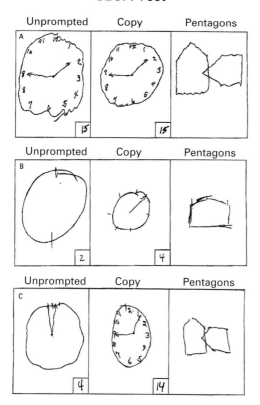

Figure 2.4 The CLOX test is designed to detect frontal lobe/executive impairment. In the first step (CLOX 1), the patient is asked to draw a freehand clock. If the patient is unable to do this or cannot do it accurately, the patient is then asked to copy a drawing of a completed clock (CLOX 2). If the first component (CLOX 1) is impaired but CLOX 2 is intact (copying ability is retained), this suggests frontal lobe/executive impairment. Reproduced from Royall *et al.* (1998), with permission from the BMJ Publishing Group.

two fundamental components: (1) an understanding of relevant facts; and (2) an appreciation of the consequences of taking or not taking a specific action. In addition to the general cognitive screen, the clinician must ask questions that are specific and relevant to each of the tasks or capacities being assessed. This always includes relevant information from key informants or caregivers. In addition to the task-specific elements of each assessment, the assessor must also carefully take into account influential 'situation-specific' factors. The same individual may be capable in a non-conflictual simple milieu, whereas he/she may be incapable if the environment becomes more complex or conflictual.

Careful documentation is required for the details of the cognitive assessment and the responses to the probing of rationale for decisions relevant to each specific capacity. The goal of this documentation is to demonstrate that the individual has both the understanding of relevant facts and the appreciation of consequences in order to conclude that the individual is indeed capable. This type of documentation, for example in making out a Will or power of attorney, will protect the patient from potential challenges to competency that may occur in the context of a conflictual family situation.

Physical examination

The high prevalence of physical illness and disability among the old renders a thorough physical examination a key element of any competent initial assessment. As well as examining the basic systems (cardiovascular, respiratory, gastrointestinal, neurological, bones and joints) for common abnormal signs (hyper- or hypotension, abnormalities of cardiac rhythm, heart failure, obstructive airways disease or areas of lung consolidation, abdominal masses (including faecal loading), hypertrophy of liver or spleen, evidence of impaired liver function (e.g. spider naevi, jaundice, etc.), focal neurological signs or evidence of Parkinsonism, examination of the fundi with an ophthalmoscope and the presence of disabling arthritis), it is vital to check eyesight and hearing and to ensure that these are optimally corrected by the use of spectacles and hearing aids where appropriate and available. If eyesight is impaired, the presence of cataracts whose removal might restore effective vision should be considered, and many old people with impaired hearing can have this improved by the use of hearing aids, although those with cognitive impairment struggle to use and not lose these pieces of equipment. Finally, the periphery should be examined. It is not uncommon to find that mobility is restricted by painful ingrowing or uncut toenails, diabetic foot disease or bunions, and Dupuytrens' contractures are not infrequent in those of Celtic descent and may impair dexterity.

Special investigations

Although we would counsel against both the blunderbuss approach of ordering every test for every patient, and the unconsidered immediate utilization of every new whiz-bang brain-imaging technique that becomes available, most elderly patients with psychiatric symptoms or apparent cognitive decline will need to undergo a basic battery of tests in order to rule out common, treatable conditions which may either be contributing to the clinical picture or else be co-morbid with it.

Tests to consider include: full blood examination (FBE) (to look for anaemias, macrocytosis, signs of response to infection and the occasional case of chronic lymphocytic leukaemia); erythrocyte sedimentation rate (a useful screen for vasculitis and some other inflammatory or malignant processes, although an equivocal result (e.g. 60 mm per hour) can prompt a wild goose chase for non-existent pathology in a very old person); B12 and folate levels (these can be low and require correction despite an apparently normal FBE); urea, electrolytes and creatinine (renal function may be impaired, especially in those with diabetes, and the frequent prescription of diuretics is commonly associated with hypokalaemia and/or hyponatraemia); calcium and phosphate (bone and parathyroid diseases may disrupt levels and correction of such abnormalities may restore a confused patient to cognitive health); liver function tests (these may pick up previously unsuspected alcohol abuse or malignant disease); random glucose (and glucose tolerance tests and/or haemoglobin A1C where diabetes mellitus is suspected or known to be present); mid-stream urine and culture (especially in females who display a recent change in cognitive function or behaviour); electrocardiogram. Some form of structural brain imaging is indicated in patients with apparent cognitive impairment, new-onset mood disorder or late-onset schizophrenia-like illness, although the yield of findings which change management from imaging will not be high. Abnormalities are most likely to be found when the history of decline is of less than one year in duration, the presenting picture is atypical for Alzheimer's disease (AD), the patient displays focal neurological signs, or is under 65 and shows cognitive impairment. For most cases a plain CT brain scan will be adequate to eliminate the possibility of tumour(s), stroke, haemorrhage, focal atrophy (e.g. in frontotemporal dementia) or hydrocephalus. When available, MRI will do more to pick up vascular disease of the brain and can be used to assess hippocampal volume which, when diminished, is a somewhat useful although not infallible guide to the presence of AD.

Other investigations to consider in certain cases include: electroencephalography (to detect epilepsy); syphilis serology and antibodies and HIV tests (in individuals or populations at risk or when symptoms suggest syphilis or HIV infection as part of the differential); lumbar puncture (when considering rare conditions such as Creuzfeldt–Jakob disease); and specialized imaging techniques such as single photon emission tomography (SPET) or positron emission tomography (PET) (although FDG and PiB PET scans are available in only a few centres around the world, and the diagnostic value of the latter type of scan is still under evaluation as we go to press). In patients with a family history of early-onset dementia, specific tests for mutations of the genes which code for presenilin 1 and/or 2, amyloid precursor protein or tau may be considered, but such patients usually will require the highly specialized services of a neurogenetics clinic and the tests are more likely to be informative when a mutation has previously been characterized in another family member. Until effective preventive treatments of AD become available, we would counsel against routine testing of apolipoprotein E status. Although the 25% of European-derived populations who carry the ε4 variant of this gene are at three times the risk of developing AD in comparison to non-carriers, the knowledge that one is ApoE ε4 positive tends to cause worry and distress and there is no effective action that can be taken to change risk status.

Referral for assessment by allied health practitioners

The availability of neuropsychologists, clinical psychologists, speech pathologists and occupational therapists varies markedly between and even within countries. Where available, neuropsychologists may assist greatly in the assessment of those with equivocal or unusual cognitive impairment, and those whose assessment is rendered more difficult by virtue of the receipt of very little or very much education, lack of fluency in the dominant language of their place of residence, or a cultural background which is very different from that of the bulk of the local population. Nobody assesses language better than a speech pathologist, and an occupational therapist's assessment of function or driving often reveals more about domestic competence, safety at home, or risk to other road users than many hours of medical assessment in the office or clinic.

Conclusion

A thorough and well-documented initial assessment is the cornerstone of competent and effective practice of the psychiatry of old age. What goes unseen goes undetected, and both the varied nature of clinical presentation and the high frequency of multiple co-morbid pathological processes in those of advanced years are powerful arguments in favour of comprehensive initial assessment.

FURTHER READING

Articles

Borson, S. *et al.* (2000). The Mini-Cog: a cognitive 'vital signs' measure for dementia screening in multi-lingual elderly. *International Journal of Geriatric Psychiatry*, **15**, 1021–1027.
A potentially useful, brief cognitive assessment instrument.

Brodaty, H. *et al.* (2002). The GPCOG: a new screening test for dementia designed for general practice. *Journal of the American Geriatrics Society*, **50**, 530–534.
Describes an increasingly popular brief assessment instrument designed for use in primary care settings.

Folstein, M. F., Folstein, S. E. and McHugh, P. R. (1975). Mini-Mental State: a practical method for grading the cognitive state of patients for the clinicians. *Journal of Psychiatric Research*, **12**, 189–198.
The archetypal brief cognitive screen.

Hodkinson, H. M. (1972). Evaluation of a mental test score for the assessment of mental impairment in the elderly. *Age and Ageing*, **1**, 233–238.
The abbreviated mental test score has the advantage of brevity, but the question about the monarch will need adaptation outside countries which belong to the British Commonwealth.

Nasreddine, Z. S. *et al.* (2005). The Montreal Cognitive Assessment, MoCA: a brief screening tool for mild cognitive impairment. *Journal of the American Geriatrics Society*, **53**, 695–699.
The MoCA is growing rapidly in popularity.

Rosen, W. G., Mohs, R. C. and Davis, K. L. (1984). A new rating scale for Alzheimer's disease. *American Journal of Psychiatry*, **141**, 1356–1364.
This paper describes the ADAS-Cog, which has been widely utilized in trials of cognitive enhancing agents. The ADAS-Cog is fairly sensitive to change and takes around 20 minutes to administer.

Roth, M. *et al.* (1984). CAMDEX: a standardised instrument for the diagnosis of mental disorder in the elderly with special reference to the early detection of dementia. *British Journal of Psychiatry*, **149**, 698–709.
The CAMDEX incorporates the CAMCOG, a mini-neuropsychological battery which assesses several areas of cognitive function. The CAMDEX can be purchased from Cambridge University Press.

Royall, D. R., Cordes, J. A. and Polk, M. (1998). CLOX: an executive clock drawing task. *Journal of Neurology Neurosurgery and Psychiatry*, **64**, 588–594.
A clock test that can help assess frontal lobe functioning.

Shulman, K. I. (2000). Clock-drawing: is it the ideal cognitive screening test? *International Journal of Geriatric Psychiatry*, **15**, 548–561.
A thorough overview.

Shulman, K. I. *et al.* (2006). IPA survey of brief cognitive screening instruments. *International Psychogeriatrics*, **18**, 281–294.
Details what instruments are in widespread use by specialists around the world.

Storey, J. E. *et al.* (2004). The Rowland Universal Dementia Assessment Scale (RUDAS): a multicultural cognitive assessment scale. *International Psychogeriatrics,* **16**, 13–31.
This instrument appears to be very good when used in the assessment of those from diverse linguistic or cultural groups, including individuals with limited formal education.

Books

David, A., Fleminger, S., Kopelman, M., Lovestone, S., and Mellers, J. (2009). *Lishman's Organic Psychiatry, 4th edition*. Chichester: Wiley.
This recently revised and updated classic text contains an excellent and very detailed section on all aspects of cognitive assessment.

Shulman, K. and Feinstein, A. (2003). *Quick Cognitive Screening for Clinicians*. London: Martin Dunitz.
A compact but comprehensive guide to this important topic.

Book chapters

Shulman, K. I. and Silver, I. L. (2006). Assessment of older adults. In D. Goldbloom, (Ed.) *Psychiatric Clinical Skills* (pp. 315–325). Philadelphia, PA: Elsevier Mosby.
A comprehensive chapter on assessment.

Silver, L. and Herrmann, N. (2004). History and mental status examination. In J. Sadavoy, L. Jarvik, G. Grossberg and B. Meyers, (Eds.) *Comprehensive Textbook of Geriatric Psychiatry*, 3rd edition (pp. 253–280). New York, NY: W.W. Norton.
Offers more detail than can be provided in the current text.

3

Differential diagnosis – the 3Ds

Introduction

This chapter addresses an approach to the differential diagnosis of the major syndromes encountered in the psychiatry of old age, namely the 3Ds – depression, delirium and dementia. In terms of prevalence, these conditions represent the vast majority of psychiatric disorders encountered in the clinical psychiatry of late life and, hence, an approach to differential diagnosis is essential in terms of understanding and management. Particular attention is given in this chapter to the relationship between depression and dementia.

History taking

Tables 3.1 and 3.2 provide a guide to the major differences in each of the 3Ds based on history and mental status examination. As reflected in the previous chapter on assessment, history taking is one of the most important means by which we establish a diagnosis and, hence, differentiate the various syndromes. Simply identifying the onset of the history of present illness (HPI) can be most revealing. Most dementing illnesses typically have an insidious, chronic and progressive course prior to the time of psychiatric assessment. Usually, this is in the order of years or at least six months in duration. The onset of illness is distinctly different in delirium in which onset in most cases is acute, developing in hours to days prior to medical attention. In between the two syndromes of dementia and delirium is major depression, whose onset tends to be sub-acute in nature, usually in the order of weeks to months. Hence, one could argue that a simple description of the timeline of the presenting symptoms can go a long way in differentiating the 3Ds and establishing a provisional diagnosis. However, as highlighted in Chapter 6, the most common risk factor for the development of delirium is dementia. Thus, one may have both a delirium and dementia as well as co-morbid depression and dementia (see below).

As often occurs, the initial assessment may not reveal an obvious provisional diagnosis and one may still be entertaining a number of clinical possibilities. In that case, simply following the patient's clinical course and monitoring outcome will frequently reveal the true nature of the underlying condition. The dementias by their very nature are degenerative conditions with a resultant progressive decline in cognition and function over time. In contrast, the course of delirium

Table 3.1 Differentiating the 3Ds in the assessment of an older adult.

	Dementia	Delirium	Depression
Onset	Insidious	Acute	Sub-acute
Course	Progressive	Increased mortality	Recovery/ recurrence
Medical status	Variable	Acute illness	Rule out medical illness
		Drug toxicity	
Family history	10% familial dementia	Negative	Mood disorder, substance abuse

Table 3.2 Differential diagnosis of psychotic symptoms.

	Dementia	Delirium	Depression
Delusions	Compensatory	Nightmarish	Nihilistic
Hallucinations	Variable	Visual	Auditory
Quality	Vacuous/banal	Frightening, bizarre	Self-deprecatory

is very different in that there is a bimodal distribution in terms of outcome. On the one hand, delirium, especially in hospitalized patients, carries a high mortality rate. However, after recovering from delirium, many patients are restored to their premorbid level of function and cognition. Recent data, however, certainly suggest that delirium is indeed a risk factor for the development of a progressive irreversible dementia.

As in mixed-age populations, the clinical course of major depression is characterized by a pattern of recovery and vulnerability to recurrence, usually with periods of relatively good functioning between episodes. However, there is of course a spectrum of those who retain persistent residual symptoms of depression. Recent studies are strongly suggestive of the fact that major depression, particularly late-onset depression, is a significant risk factor for the development of an irreversible dementia. Even the presence of depressive symptoms may be predictive of an increased risk for developing dementia when patients are followed over several years. The incidence of dementia is almost always significantly greater in those with a history of depression compared to those without any depressive history.

Associated with depression and delirium is a condition that has been known as 'pseudodementia' or 'reversible dementia'. This has been defined as a clinical condition in which the presence of transient cognitive impairment is associated with a depressive syndrome. One must ensure that at the time of the cognitive impairment, there is no evidence of an obvious neuropathological process that can explain the cognitive change which is usually attributed to the depressive illness itself. The transient nature of the cognitive impairment is considered a result of the treatment of the underlying depressive illness, hence, the term 'pseudodementia'. However, several studies which have followed pseudodementia patients over a longer timeframe reveal the disconcerting evidence that these patients are also subject to the development of irreversible dementias. Indeed, the longer the follow-up, the greater the proportion of pseudodementia patients that eventually become demented. Figures 3.1–3.3 are illustrative of the relationship between depression, dementia and reversible dementias reflecting the prevalence of co-morbidities and the shift over time from depressive syndromes to dementia. Early studies involving relatively short follow-up trials of one to two years did not reveal the apparent vulnerability to developing dementia that has become more evident with longer-term outcome studies.

Medical history

The understanding of medical co-morbidity is an important feature that distinguishes the understanding and management of psychiatric disorders in later life from mixed-age populations. For the dementias, the medical status can be extremely variable, ranging from severely ill bedridden individuals to those who appear to be perfectly healthy, robust and independent from a physical perspective yet are dependent on others for independent activities of daily living.

For delirium, on the other hand, an acute medical illness, by definition, has overwhelmed the central nervous system, and hence the identification of delirium suggests that such patients should be carefully assessed by a medical practitioner. Specifically, attention to drug toxicity and drug interactions is a vitally important aspect of the assessment of the syndrome of delirium. Drugs with anticholinergic properties are particularly deliriogenic.

In major depression, the relationship to underlying medical illness is also important. This is especially so in refractory depressions that do not respond to usual psychiatric treatments. A negative family history of mood disorder and negative past psychiatric history should raise the index of suspicion that there is an underlying systemic medical illness, such as a carcinoma or neurologic condition that is producing the depressive syndrome.

Family history

Family history remains an important clue to differential diagnosis. Commonly, a referral for a psychogeriatric consultation asks to distinguish between a mood disorder and a developing dementia. In its early stages, dementing illnesses may not be evident and, given what we know about depression as a risk factor for dementia, this becomes an important clinical challenge. As in mixed-age populations and especially younger adults, major depression still is associated with a significant familial or genetic vulnerability. This is less so in late-onset depressions

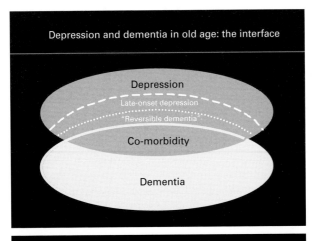

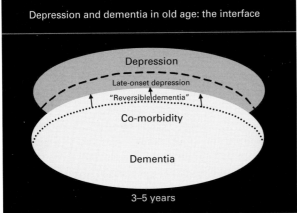

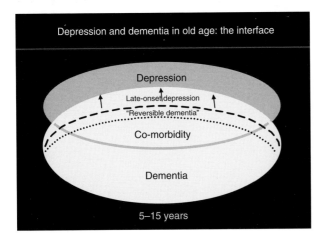

Figures 3.1–3.3 These figures illustrate the relationship between depression, dementia and reversible dementias, reflecting the prevalence of co-morbidities and the shift over time from depressive syndromes to dementia. Reproduced with permission from Shulman, K. I. and Silver, I. L. (2006). Assessment of older adults. In D. Goldbloom, (Ed.) *Psychiatric Clinical Skills* (pp. 315–325). Philadelphia, PA: Elsevier Mosby.

of older adults where medical and neurological factors command greater significance. However, when a clinician needs to make a decision as to whether to treat a questionable depressive illness, the presence of a family history may be the one factor that tips the balance in favour of a trial of antidepressant therapy. Dementias on the other hand also have a familial propensity, particularly those with early-onset Alzheimer's disease (AD). Thus, the presence of a family history of dementia, as opposed to mood disorders, may shift the weight of evidence in the direction of one syndrome compared to another.

Given recent data, the presence of a family history of mood disorder and indeed a past history of mood disorder does not protect the individual from the increased risk of ultimately developing a dementing illness over time, and indeed the possibility of both syndromes being present needs to be considered. As a general rule, even when there is evidence of dementia or cognitive impairment, the presence of a persistent and clinically significant depressive syndrome usually invites treatment of depression in its own right.

False theories of depression and dementia

It may be worthwhile to review a number of theories about the relationship of depression and dementia that have proven to be false although at first glance they may appear to have intuitive merit.

1. Hypothesis: major depression in later life is primarily due to the losses associated with old age.

Clinical experience suggests that it is the losses in early life that may be more relevant to the risk of developing a depressive illness later in life. Early losses and traumas contribute to vulnerable personalities which may in turn be overwhelmed by the stressors of late life (medical and psychological stressors). It is important to remember that the vast majority of older people cope with the vicissitudes of later life, which include multiple losses, without developing a major depression.

2. Hypothesis: depression, delirium and dementia are distinct syndromes.

The previous section summarized the evidence for a relationship between the '3Ds'. They are not as distinct as originally postulated, especially when one looks at clinical outcome, an important feature of psychiatric illnesses. Hence, the presence of delirium and major depression in later life do seem to create an increased vulnerability to the development of irreversible dementias over time. Conversely, dementia is associated with an increased risk of depression and delirium.

3. Hypothesis: subjective cognitive impairment or complaints of memory impairment are associated with depression.

This was the original teaching of the geriatric psychiatrists who began describing late-life psychiatric syndromes. It was felt that the complaints of subjective memory impairment were reflective of depressive illnesses. However, once again, long-term outcome studies have refuted this hypothesis and subjective memory impairment is, in a significant proportion of cases, a prodrome of a developing dementia. Similarly, mild cognitive impairment (MCI) (see Chapter 4), or what was termed 'benign senescent forgetfulness' by V.A. Kral, may not be benign in many cases. Like subjective complaints of cognitive impairment, MCI can be a forerunner of a developing dementia.

4. Hypothesis: the use of antidepressants with marked anticholinergic properties may be the cause of dementia.

This was another interesting theory advocated by V. A. Kral. Given the cholinergic hypothesis of dementia (i.e. a cholinergic deficit), this seemed to be a plausible theory, but once again the evidence does not support the suggestion that antidepressants aggravate the development of dementia. Although this should not be a reason to withhold antidepressant treatment from those who are affected by both depression and dementia, it should be noted that recently developed classes of antidepressant are not as anticholinergic as the original tricyclics and it should therefore be possible to avoid exposing most people with dementia to antidepressant drugs with the potential to affect cholinergic function adversely.

5. Hypothesis: depression is a psychological reaction to impaired cognition.

Patients who are aware of their failing cognition may be understandably distressed. However, the evidence that the subjective awareness of cognitive change leads to a major depression without other risk factors for depression has not been forthcoming. Some have even suggested that there may be a neurobiological substrate for 'reactive' depression.

Evidence-based hypotheses of a relationship between depression and dementia

A number of theories have tried to explain the evidence that depression can be a forerunner of dementia in later life. One theory suggests that both depression and dementia have shared risk factors. In particular, vascular disease may be related to the aetiology of 'vascular depression' as well as the development of 'vascular cognitive impairment' or 'vascular dementia'. The vascular depression hypothesis is based on the association of vascular disease and vascular risk factors with depression in late life. Moreover, the vascular depression subtype appears to be associated with more cognitive dysfunction than non-vascular depression and relatively more disability for the same level of depression. These individuals also tend to lack insight into their illness and demonstrate low levels of pure depressive ideation, such as guilt or morbid preoccupations with death and suicide.

Both late-life depression and dementia have been associated with atrophy of the left hippocampus. Recent work has suggested that a reduction in hippocampal volume may be related to the total duration time of major depression found in women. Having a history of depression was also associated with smaller hippocampal volumes bilaterally. Smaller hippocampal volumes have recently been confirmed in older depressive subjects compared to controls. An extension of this work examined the association of small left hippocampal volume with an increased risk of dementia. Indeed, there seems to be an increased incidence of dementia in depressed patients who have smaller left hippocampal volumes but have not yet met criteria for the diagnosis of dementia. Thus, this neuroanatomic region may be a factor in the close relationship of depression and dementia.

Another link between hippocampus size, depression and dementia was postulated by the Australian psychologist Tony Jorm, building on work by the American neurophysiologist, Robert Sapolsky. This is based on the hypothesis that stress may result in an increased secretion of glucocorticoids from the adrenal glands. The hippocampus contains glucocorticoid receptors that could play a role in inhibiting further secretion of glucocorticoids. However, degeneration of the hippocampus in both depression and dementia may cause an impairment in glucocorticoid feedback inhibition. In turn, excess and continuous secretion of glucocorticoids may damage the hippocampus, causing further impairment. This 'glucocorticoid cascade hypothesis' may provide a neurobiological basis for the linkage between depression and dementia.

Jorm takes seriously the evidence that depression may indeed be a risk factor for developing progressive cognitive decline. However, he rightly points out that the size of that association is relatively small, so that very large sample sizes may be required to demonstrate this association. This is best done through epidemiologic studies rather than clinical samples.

Clinical implications of the growing relationship between depression and dementia

The finding of an increased risk of progressive irreversible cognitive change associated with depressive illnesses in older adults suggests a number of clinical implications. The first is increased vigilance for cognitive change in those with major depressions in late life, especially those with a late-onset depression. Additional vigilance should be conferred on those who have a family history of dementia in first-degree relatives or those who at initial assessment have evidence of MCI or have persistent and prominent subjective complaints of memory impairment or dysfunction. In those patients with an increased risk and where increased vigilance is suggested, neuroimaging may be helpful in diagnosis or at least establishing a baseline for future reference. Certainly, regular screening using brief cognitive instruments will be useful in detecting change. In addition, regular input from carers/informants remains essential in identifying intellectual, affective and behavioural changes associated with a developing dementia.

Notwithstanding the increased risk of dementia, the presence of a persistent and prominent depressive syndrome does invite specific antidepressant treatment. If the glucocorticoid cascade hypothesis turns out to be correct then, indeed, there will be a neurobiological rationale for aggressively treating depression and having a protective effect on degeneration of the left hippocampus. None the less, even without a validated theory, concern for quality of life does suggest that treating clinically significant symptoms of depression is a worthwhile enterprise as long as it is done in a carefully monitored fashion.

Finally, the association with vascular disease suggests that, from a medical perspective, there should be an optimization of vascular risk factors including management of hypertension, diabetes, hyperlipidaemias and cholesterol levels as well as stroke prevention. Particular attention must be paid to those suffering from atrial fibrillation where embolic phenomena may be contributory to a variety of neuropsychiatric syndromes.

FURTHER READING

Articles

Alexopoulos, G. S. *et al.* (1993). The course of geriatric depression with 'reversible dementia': a controlled study. *American Journal of Psychiatry,* **150**, 1693–1699.
A classic follow-up study of patients with what was once termed 'depressive pseudodementia'.

Baldwin, R. C. and O'Brien, J. (2002). Vascular basis of late-onset depressive disorder. *British Journal of Psychiatry,* **180**, 157–160.
A thoughtful review of the relationship between cerebrovascular disease and depression.

Jorm, A. F. (2000). Is depression a risk factor for dementia or cognitive decline? *Gerontology,* 46, 219–227.
A thorough consideration of evidence for and against the idea that depression predisposes to cognitive decline.

Book chapter

Shulman, K. I. and Silver, I. L. (2006). Assessment of older adults. In D. Goldbloom, (Ed.) *Psychiatric Clinical Skills* (pp. 315–325). Philadelphia, PA: Elsevier Mosby.
Recommended reading for all aspiring old age psychiatrists and geriatricians.

4

The dementias

Defining dementia

Definitions of dementia have been getting progressively longer and more complex. Fifty years ago, a leading psychiatric textbook defined dementia in one short sentence. Now, diagnostic manuals devote pages to its definition. Tables 4.1 and 4.2 give summaries of the diagnostic criteria used by the World Health Organization's ICD-10 and the American Psychiatric Association's DSM-IV-TR systems, which are the criteria most used in clinical practice and research today. It should be noted that strict application of these different criteria will yield different rates of dementia in any population assessed, because the criteria differ in the levels of impairment required to diagnose dementia. However, all definitions of dementia include certain core features. First, dementia is a *syndrome* (a collection of symptoms and signs) with multiple causes. Second, dementia is an *acquired* condition and represents a *decline* from a previous level of function no matter how exalted or limited that level of function used to be. Third, the diagnosis can be made only in an *alert* patient, because the main differential diagnosis is delirium, which is characterized by both cognitive impairment and an impaired level of consciousness. Fourth, while memory impairment is a necessary feature of the disorder, dementia affects not only memory but *multiple* higher mental functions such as intellect and personality. Finally, dementia is not a diagnosis based solely on the patient's performance in an unfamiliar clinical setting, but must be rooted in real-world problems: namely, impairment of *social or occupational functioning.* Reversible dementia syndromes exist and some dementias can present with static impairments that do not get worse, but most cases of dementia are irreversible and progressive.

Types and causes of dementia

Table 4.3 lists a large number of causes of dementia, including conditions that may present with an apparent dementia syndrome. However, most such presentations are not frequently encountered in clinical practice. Alzheimer's disease (AD), vascular dementia (VaD), mixed vascular and Alzheimer's disease, dementia with Lewy bodies (DLB), frontotemporal dementias (FTD) and dementia associated with alcohol abuse are the commonest types of dementia seen.

Table 4.1 ICD-10 diagnostic criteria for dementia (abbreviated).

G1. There is evidence of each of the following:
 1. A decline in memory, most evident in the learning of new information. The decline should be verified by a reliable history from an informant, supplemented, if possible, by neuropsychological tests or quantified cognitive assessments.
 2. A decline in other cognitive abilities characterized by deterioration in judgement and thinking, such as planning and organizing, and in the general processing of information. Evidence should be obtained from an informant and supplemented, if possible, by neuropsychological tests or quantified objective assessments. Deterioration from a previously higher level of performance should be established.
G2. Awareness of the environment is preserved sufficiently long to allow the unequivocal demonstration of the symptoms in criterion G1.
G3. There is decline in emotional control or motivation, or a change in social behaviour manifested as at least one of:
 1. emotional lability
 2. irritability
 3. apathy
 4. coarsening of social behaviour.
G4. For a confident diagnosis, the symptoms in criterion G1 should have been present for at least six months.
The full criteria specify the levels of impairment in both criteria G1 and G2 characteristic of mild, moderate and severe dementia and suggest categorizing cases according to cause (e.g. Alzheimer's disease, vascular dementia, etc.) and the presence or absence of additional symptoms.

Adapted from World Health Organization. (1993). *The ICD-10 Classification of Mental and Behavioural Disorders.* Geneva: WHO. ISBN 92 4 154455 4.
Readers should refer to the original document for the full criteria.

Alzheimer's disease

First described over 100 years ago, AD is a progressive neurodegenerative disorder characterized by the presence of amyloid plaques between cortical neurones and neurofibrillary tangles within them. The occipital and motor cortices are relatively spared, while the lesions and associated atrophy tend to develop first in the entorhinal cortex and hippocampus before spreading throughout the temporal, parietal and frontal lobes. The plaques are aggregations of insoluble amyloid $A\beta42$ protein, a breakdown product of amyloid precursor protein (APP), a ubiquitous normal protein that may have a role in cell surface membrane reception. The tangles are comprised of hyperphosphorylated tau protein and represent the damaged remains of neurotubules which are essential for the transport of nutrients to the extensive dendrites and axons of these neurones. In AD, a slow cascade of events occurring over up to three decades leads to damage to dendritic connections and death of neurones. Although the disease process is asymptomatic in its early years, ultimately this damage destroys enough cellular connections

Table 4.2 DSM-IV-TR criteria for dementia (abbreviated).

A. The development of multiple cognitive deficits manifested by both:
   1. Memory impairment
   2. One or more of:
      a) aphasia
      b) apraxia
      c) agnosia
      d) disturbance in executive functioning.
B. The cognitive deficits in criterion A1 and A2 EACH cause significant impairment in social and occupational functioning and represent a significant decline from a previous level of functioning.
C. The characteristics and course of the disorder are defined separately for each type of dementia (Alzheimer's disease, vascular dementia, dementia due to other medical conditions, substance-induced dementia, dementia due to multiple aetiologies, dementia not otherwise specified) as are those conditions other than dementia which can produce cognitive impairment and thereby exclude the diagnosis of dementia (e.g. delirium, major depression, etc.).

Other symptoms, the presence or absence of co-morbid behavioural disturbance and onset before or after 65 years of age all may be classified in this diagnostic system.

Note: DSM-IV-TR has separate criteria for the six types of dementia listed at criterion C and only those features common to all definitions have been tabulated here. The reader should refer to the original document for the full criteria.
Adapted from American Psychiatric Association. (2000). *Quick Reference to the Diagnostic Criteria from DSM-IV-TR*. Washington, DC: American Psychiatric Association. ISBN 0–89042–026–2.

to produce the characteristic symptoms of impaired new learning, dyspraxia, dysphasia, loss of judgement and, eventually, the complete loss of higher mental functions and the utter dependency of the affected individual. Death results from pneumonia associated with debility if no other co-morbid disease process claims the life of the affected patient before this stage is reached.

Although some uncertainties about the nature of the pathological processes driving AD remain, it appears that the amyloid protein produced from APP plays a key role in initiating inflammatory processes that damage neurones and set off the accumulation of tangles and progressive neuronal loss.

Depending on the exact diagnostic criteria used, AD accounts for, or is a major contributory cause in, between 50 and 80% of all dementias. The main risk factors for AD are advancing age, a family history of AD and the possession of the ε4 allele of the lipid transport protein apolipoprotein E (ApoE). Rare mutations in the APP gene on chromosome 21, the presenilin 1 gene on chromosome 14 and the presenilin 2 gene on chromosome 1 are causative of dominantly inherited familial AD with onset between age 40 and 60. Although these familial dementias account for only 1% of all AD, the fact that these genes all produce proteins with a key role in the production of Aβ42 amyloid is a key piece of evidence in support of the 'amyloid hypothesis' of AD causation.

Table 4.3 Causes of the dementia syndrome.

Neurodegenerative
Alzheimer's disease
Dementia with Lewy bodies
Parkinson's disease
Frontal and frontotemporal dementias
Vascular
Infarction(s)
Haemorrhage
Cardiovascular disease
Binswanger's encephalopathy
Vasculitis
Endocrine disorders
Diabetes
Hypo- or hyperthyroidism
Parathyroid disease
Cushing's disease
Addison's disease
Vitamin deficiencies
B12, thiamine (B1) and nicotinic acid
Systemic diseases
Severe respiratory disease
Anaemia
Other disorders of metabolism
Hyper- or hypocalcaemia
Severe liver disease
Neurological disorders and trauma
'Normal pressure' hydrocephalus
Head injury
Space-occupying lesions (e.g. tumours, haematomas)
Multiple sclerosis
Infections
Syphilis
Viral encephalitis
HIV
Creutzfeldt–Jakob disease
Substance use, abuse or withdrawal
Drugs
Alcohol
Psychiatric syndromes
Severe depression
Mania
 Schizophrenia

Vascular dementia

A variety of manifestations of cerebrovascular disease, ranging from a large cortical infarction to multiple small infarcts, down to subtle white matter changes due to small vessel ischaemia and resultant hypoperfusion, can produce a dementia syndrome. The symptoms of dementia seen in people with cerebrovascular disease depend on the nature of the underlying damage, but often frontal features such as lack of initiative are prominent, as are mood symptoms, especially depressed mood. Deficits tend to be patchy and unequal, onset is usually abrupt, and progression is more likely to be stepwise or intermittent rather than steady or inexorable. Diagnostic criteria for VaD emphasize the presence of focal neurological signs (which may be transient), the presence of infarction in structural images obtained with CT or MRI and/or the presence of significant white matter changes affecting at least 25% of the white matter.

Mixed vascular and Alzheimer dementia

In autopsy series, the presence of at least some degree of cerebrovascular disease is common in the brains of those diagnosed as having AD during life. In addition, at least some pathological changes typical of AD are found in the brains of over 90% of VaD patients who undergo a post-mortem brain examination. The fact that vascular risk factors such as hypertension, diabetes, hypercholesterolaemia, smoking, obesity and lack of exercise are associated with both VaD and AD in some studies may be due to these factors having some direct effect on APP metabolism, or could suggest that subtle cerebrovascular arteriosclerosis can ensure that the symptomatic phase of AD is manifest earlier in those with AD pathology that might not yet be sufficient to produce cognitive impairment on its own.

Dementia with Lewy bodies

Early in the twentieth century, Friedrich Lewy described inclusion bodies in the neurones of the brain stem of individuals affected by Parkinson's disease. In the early 1990s, the microscopic examination of the cortical regions of some patients with primary progressive dementias revealed the presence of ubiquitin staining Lewy bodies in these regions too. Retrospective analysis of case records and subsequent prospective research indicated that individuals with primary progressive dementias who manifest any two of markedly fluctuating cognitive impairments, spontaneous motor Parkinsonism and/or visual hallucinations in clear consciousness, are highly likely to exhibit cortical Lewy bodies at autopsy. Such patients usually are exquisitely sensitive to the extra-pyramidal side effects of antipsychotic drugs. It seems likely that DLB sits on a disease spectrum with Parkinson's disease and that the initial symptomatic manifestation of the underlying pathology may be either motor or cognitive, depending on the distribution of the lesions that characterize these conditions.

Frontotemporal dementias

A wide spectrum of pathologies producing progressive dementias that affect primarily the frontal lobes has been described. The clinical presentation will vary according to the main initial focus of degeneration in the brain. Illnesses that attack the inferior frontal lobes tend to present with disinhibited behaviours which cause embarrassment to others and may put the person with dementia at risk of injury or assault. Judgement is usually poor in these cases, often endangering others as well as the patient (e.g. from dangerous driving). Posterior frontal lobe damage may result in semantic difficulties and progressive aphasias. As frontal dementias progress, apathy, produced by damage to the motivation centres in the interhemispheric fissure, becomes the most prominent feature of the illness until almost complete inanition supervenes.

Between one-third and one-half of frontal dementias are familial illnesses with a dominant pattern of inheritance. Mutations in the tau protein gene on chromosome 14 account for some but not all of these cases.

Frontal dementias tend to come on earlier than AD, with most cases manifesting in the sixth or seventh decade of life.

Dementias associated with alcohol abuse

End-organ vulnerability to the adverse effects of chronic overconsumption of alcohol varies markedly between individuals in respect of the liver and heart and the same is true of the brain. Lack of thiamine is a key mechanism in damage to the brain associated with over-use of alcohol, although the extent to which alcohol produces direct neurotoxicity remains controversial. Typically temporal (memory) and frontal functions are affected to the greatest degree in dementias associated with alcohol.

Other uncommon dementias

For detailed descriptions of uncommon dementias, the reader is referred to the list of further reading at the chapter's end. Dementia associated with syphilis, once very common, is now rare and tends to be characterized by disinhibition. Dementia associated with AIDS tends to be a late manifestation of infection with HIV and most AIDS dementia patients do not live for very long.

Mild cognitive impairment

Mild cognitive impairment (MCI) is a term coined by North American researchers keen to identify people at high risk of developing AD before the impairments of function required to diagnose dementia are present. The concept is not new, and earlier terms such as 'cognitive impairment not dementia' (CIND) and 'age-associated memory impairment' (AAMI) will be encountered in the literature and sometimes in clinical practice. The ICD-10 diagnostic category of mild cognitive disorder also derives from the historical concept of AAMI and other related ideas. Use of the term MCI by clinicians is increasing, as they see more and more such patients in clinical settings as the population ages and awareness of the treatability of some forms of dementia grows. MCI is defined arbitrarily as performance 1.5 standard deviations below the age- and education-adjusted norm on at least one neuropsychological test, where activities of daily living are substantially unimpaired, and either the person with the memory problem or a close relative is aware of and bothered by the difficulty. Amnestic (affecting memory alone), non-amnestic and multi-domain forms of MCI have been described. Although no treatments have yet been proven to help this condition, subjects diagnosed with MCI should be followed regularly, as up to 15% (depending on the diagnostic criteria used and the population from which the individuals are drawn) will develop AD with each year that passes, though one-third never decline in this way. Several strategies that may help people with MCI are being actively researched and include cognitive retraining, exercise and some drug therapies.

The epidemiology of dementia

Dementia is extremely common and becoming ever more so. The reason for this is simple. Dementia is an age-related disorder and the chances of being affected by dementia double every five years between the ages of 60 and 90. It is expected that there will be 40 million people with dementia in the world by 2020 and over 80 million by 2040 (see Chapter 1). The majority of these people will live in developing countries. All societies, races and cultures that have been studied have been found to contain people with dementia, but comparative epidemiology has not yet determined with any surety whether people living in one country or people derived from particular parts of the world are especially at risk of or uniquely protected against dementia.

The main risk factors for dementia are age, family history of dementia, the possession of one or more ApoE ε4 alleles (which trebles the risk of dementia developing at any age), a head injury with post-traumatic amnesia exceeding one hour, and female sex. Vascular risk factors (hypertension, diabetes, obesity, hypercholesterolaemia, smoking) appear to increase the risk of not only vascular dementia but also AD. While most dementias manifest in late life, a small but important minority of people develop dementia in mid-adulthood and their needs and problems are often quite different from those of elderly people with dementia. More than half of such early-onset cases carry rare genetic mutations (usually dominantly inherited) which are causative of early-onset dementia, including mutations in genes which affect APP processing (leading to early-onset AD) and the tau gene (which can lead to early-onset FTD). Although dominantly inherited dementias account for only about 1% of all dementias, specialist genetic counselling and testing services are required to assist both affected and unaffected members of such families. Services for people with early-onset dementia need to cater for a very vulnerable group of patients, whose families are especially stressed by the decline of a family member in what should be the very prime of life. Such services should be distinct from generic services for late-onset dementias, and are best organized at a regional level because of the relatively small number of such patients in any one area.

The symptoms and natural history of dementia

Mild

Although the initial and subsequent symptoms of dementia will depend upon the nature of the underlying disease process causing it, the majority of cases are due to AD so the symptoms of this illness will form the basis for the descriptions in this section.

Historically, most people diagnosed with dementia present because their relatives are concerned rather than because they themselves have insight into their deficits, although this may be changing with increased awareness of both dementia and the fact that some forms are treatable. Forgetfulness of recent events, missing appointments, diminishing ability to manage one's affairs and some degree of social withdrawal and declining motivation are common early features. Sometimes a person with dementia presents soon after their spouse, who had been assisting the person to a greater extent than others had realized, has left the scene due to death or illness.

Assessment of those with mild dementia usually reveals rapid forgetting of newly learned information and may also detect mild nominal dysphasia, dyscalculia, constructional dyspraxia, rigidity of thought and some impairment of judgement. Progression tends to be slow, and if the affected individual receives a cognitive enhancer there may be some months of improved performance before deterioration resumes and the individual reverts to and then passes their initial baseline. The phase of mild dementia may last for months or years, but in the typical 10-year course of an average case of AD, from two to five years is likely to be spent in this phase of illness.

A mildly demented person can be left alone safely for hours at a time, and some manage alone at home with support. Getting lost in familiar places is unusual when dementia is mild, and sometimes driving ability is retained in the early months of dementia. Although less attention may be paid to keeping one's person and home neat and tidy than was formerly the case, people with mild dementia can bathe, dress and use the lavatory without assistance. More complex activities such as handling finances or engaging in paid employment tend to be impaired at this stage.

Moderate

Whereas a mildly demented person may appear unimpaired to a casual observer, the fact that impairments are present is readily apparent soon after meeting someone with moderate dementia. Household tasks, medication use and finances will need to be managed by a family member or friend. Some difficulties with dressing may be apparent, especially in regard to the use of catches, zips and buttons, and clothes will not be changed without prompting. Bathing will need to be prompted and may require direct supervision. Inappropriate, disturbed and disturbing behaviours are common (see Chapter 5) and the patient cannot be left unsupervised for more than a few minutes. Some family members may no longer be recognized, although some personal information and the sense of self are likely to be retained. This phase may last from one to five years.

Severe

The patient with severe dementia is dependent upon others for even basic activities such as dressing, bathing, toileting and often eating as well. Continence is lost, language is restricted or lost altogether, and constant supervision is required. In the final stages of dementia, mobility is lost and unless preventive action is taken contractures and bedsores may develop. Many people with dementia die of vascular disease and cancers, but deaths due to both accidents and pneumonia are more common in those with dementia than among the rest of the population. Although severely demented people who are cared for well sometimes live for up to a decade, death from pneumonia usually occurs within one to three years.

Assessment and diagnosis

All too often, dementia presents late in the course of the disorder when valuable opportunities to prevent crises and forestall entry to residential care have been lost. Early referral to specialist services should be encouraged and such services must be equipped to diagnose and manage mild dementia as well as more advanced cases.

Although this section will describe some of the specific features of an assessment aimed at determining the presence or absence of a dementia syndrome, the reader is referred to Chapters 2 and 3 for additional information on this topic.

Informant history

Although some people with early dementia present to doctors with concerns about their memory, in most cases it is family members who initiate the process of assessment and diagnosis. The most important element of the initial assessment is obtaining a history from an informant who knows the patient well. If the patient and informant are to be seen by the same practitioner then it shows greater respect to the patient if the informant interview takes place second. However, in many specialist clinics an informant interview is undertaken by a nurse or allied health professional while a medical practitioner sees the patient. Although the patient's permission should be sought, the best way to conclude the initial consultation is to give some feedback about the findings of the assessment both to the patient and to the person(s) who accompany them to the consultation together.

In the informant interview it is important to allow time for the story to emerge and the interviewee to explain the situation and to raise areas of concern, but some formal questioning will almost certainly be necessary. The nature and extent of any cognitive deficits together with information about their impact on the patient's life should be determined. Any difficulties in everyday life such as getting lost, problems managing medications, finances and shopping should be enquired about. If the patient drives the informant's opinion of their driving competence should be sought – 'Would you let your children drive with him/her?' is sometimes a useful question. Financial competence and whether the patient has a current Will and/or an enduring power of attorney in place should be determined. As well as information about past medical history and current medications, any family history of dementia needs to be elicited. Behavioural and psychological symptoms of dementia form a separate chapter of this book, but they must be routinely enquired about at the initial informant interview. Finally, because stress, distress, depression and anxiety are common in the carers of those who have dementia, gentle enquiry as to the effect of the patient's symptoms upon the informant and how the informant is feeling about and managing the situation is an essential component of this assessment.

Medical assessment

A history about the presenting complaint should be elicited from the patient, although quite often a profound lack of insight about some or all of the many problems in living that the patient is encountering will mean that the patient does not see why they need to be assessed. In these circumstances tact, compassion and diplomacy are required! Detailed personal and family histories should be obtained in addition to past and current medical history.

Screening for depressive and anxiety symptoms may be done with a standard questionnaire or by direct probing. Cognitive assessment should utilize at least one standard screening instrument such as the Mini-mental State Examination, GPCOG, Mini-Cog or Abbreviated Mental Test Score. Depending on what is found, such tests may well need to be supplemented with additional tests of memory (e.g. sentence recall, general knowledge), language function, praxis and frontal function. Sometimes, especially when no neuropsychologist is available, a longer cognitive assessment instrument such as the ADAS-Cog or CAMCOG may be utilized. References for these and other useful cognitive assessment instruments are provided at the end of Chapter 2.

It is essential to review all current prescribed medications with a particular emphasis on those that may depress CNS function or which have anticholinergic properties.

Physical examination should be thorough and must include the cardiovascular, respiratory, gastrointestinal and neurological components. Many people with dementia have co-morbid medical conditions and sometimes these have not been diagnosed before and/or are not receiving appropriate treatment.

Neuropsychological tests

Assessment by a trained neuropsychologist can be invaluable when the cognitive impairment is mild or does not conform to an expected pattern, especially when the patient is younger than most. A neuropsychological assessment can take anything from one to three hours and will utilize standard tests appropriate for assessment of any deficits the patient may manifest. Not all patients with dementia need to be seen by a neuropsychologist, but it is very hard to offer a comprehensive dementia and cognitive assessment service if no neuropsychologist is available.

Special investigations

It is more common to detect treatable co-morbid disease than to find a reversible cause for dementia when special tests are ordered. These days, many of the investigations listed below will have been performed by a general practitiones (GP) before the patient arrives for specialist assessment and it is important that duplication of tests be avoided for reasons of cost and patient discomfort.

Most specialists would request full blood examination (to rule out anaemia and rarer blood disorders), B12 and folate levels (most deficiencies found will be mild and will not be the main cause of the cognitive impairment, but should be treated to prevent future problems), erythrocyte sedimentation rate (some dementias are caused by vasculopathies), liver function tests (these may reveal hitherto unsuspected alcohol abuse), electrolytes, creatinine and urea (to rule out renal impairment), thyroid-stimulating hormone (thyroid disease is common in late life), glucose (and HbA1C in known diabetics), and we would advocate measuring calcium and phosphate as well.

An ECG should be performed, especially if prescription of a cholinesterase inhibitor is contemplated, as heart block should be corrected before conduction is slowed further by prescription of a cholinergic drug.

It is uncommon for the results of structural neuroimaging to lead to a change in management, but in most developed countries a plain CT scan or an MRI scan will be ordered to determine the extent of any cerebrovascular pathology, to rule out space-occupying lesions and to look for supportive evidence for the putative diagnosis such as generalized or focal cerebral atrophy. Sometimes a scan can be used as an educational tool to assist the patient's family in understanding the organic nature of the changes they have observed in their affected relative (e.g. relating cerebral atrophy to decline in performance).

The use of more specialized tests such as syphilis serology and autoantibody tests, SPET brain scan or EEG can be reserved for cases where their use is specifically indicated. More specialized imaging techniques such as PET or functional magnetic resonance imaging (fMRI) are, at present, research tools rather than aids to the routine diagnostic process.

Managing the person with dementia and their carers

Imparting the diagnosis

Telling someone that they have dementia is a huge responsibility and it should be done with compassion, honesty and sufficient time available to answer questions and to discuss the implications. As most people with dementia have family or friends who will end up providing some care to them, and because it is common for family members rather than people with dementia to urge them to attend for assessment, the preferred method of imparting the diagnosis is in the setting of a family meeting in which both the patient and significant others (e.g. spouse, children) are present.

Although honesty is important, hope should not be extinguished. Some treatments are helpful in some dementias and all people with dementia have the potential to benefit from social support and education of their families.

Some of the issues that need to be addressed include the precise diagnosis, its prognosis and the potential benefits and risks of any treatment. Driving should be discussed at an early stage (most people with dementia who wish to continue to drive will need a formal driving assessment) and issues such as Wills and power of attorney should be discussed. Most countries now have Alzheimer associations or societies which provide advice, support and education to people with dementia and their carers and provision of contact details and encouragement to get in touch with the local association should be a key outcome of this interview.

Like other devastating diseases, the imparting of a dementia diagnosis may cause distress that may make it hard for the recipient of the diagnosis and their family to remember all that has been discussed. For this reason the provision of written feedback is essential and in routine practice it is common for questions and discussion about the diagnosis, prognosis and management strategies to form the topic of an ongoing dialogue between patient, family and the treating team of many months or years.

Although many GPs take a strong interest in dementia and are highly competent in its management, in most countries it is likely that the initial diagnosis will be made in a specialist setting, with some or all of the ongoing responsibility for management reverting to the GP after that has been done. It is helpful to both patient and family if specialists remain available for future consultation and advice after the initial diagnosis has been made and the management plan decided upon. Such availability also assists with the education of GPs, many of whom have received limited formal education about dementia.

Co-morbid medical conditions

It is important that co-morbid medical conditions, whether diagnosed previously, or at the time of the dementia assessment, be optimally managed by the patient's GP and any medical specialists involved with care. In particular, vascular risk factors should be managed assertively in case any contribution to the dementia is being made by vascular disease. Previously prescribed and any new medications will need to be supervised by a responsible person and the use of a dosette box or Webster pack is recommended.

Drug treatments

Most of the drug treatments for dementia were designed to treat AD, although some patients whose dementia has a vascular element may also benefit from their use.

Cholinesterase inhibitors

People with AD and DLB are likely to benefit from the prescription of a cholinesterase inhibitor, although not all will be helped and some are unable to tolerate the drugs. In many, but not all, developed countries, the cost of these medications is subsidized by insurance schemes or direct government support. Tacrine has been superseded by less toxic drugs, and the three currently in use are donepezil, galantamine and rivastigmine. There is no convincing evidence that any one of these drugs is superior in efficacy to the other two, although there is some suggestion from trials that the latter two may be less well tolerated than donepezil at the upper end of their dosage range. In practice, the choice of drug may hinge upon the mode of administration (see below), the dosage schedule or the prescribing practitioner's experience.

All cholinesterase inhibitors have the potential to produce gastrointestinal side effects, especially anorexia, nausea, vomiting, diarrhoea and abdominal discomfort. They tend to slow heart rate and may precipitate heart block in vulnerable individuals. Nightmares sometimes occur when cholinesterase inhibitors are prescribed, and these seem to be commonest when donepezil is used.

Donepezil is available as 5 and 10 mg tablets. It is usually given at night to diminish the likelihood of nausea, but many patients tolerate morning administration quite well. The starting dose is 5 mg daily increasing to 10 mg daily after 4 weeks. If the 10 mg dose is not tolerated, reversion to 5 mg per day may still be associated with some benefit.

Galantamine is sold as a slow-release capsule given once each day. The initial dose is 8 mg daily for one month and then 16 mg per day, increasing to 24 mg if no improvement is seen or when later deterioration becomes manifest.

Rivastigmine is manufactured in capsules, as a liquid and in the form of a skin patch. The capsules and liquid (the latter useful for those who cannot swallow easily) need to be given at least twice daily because of the drug's relatively short half-life, but the patch can be applied once every 24 hours and left in place until the next one is due. Oral administration commences with 1.5 mg twice daily and aims to reach 6 mg twice daily after two months with 3 mg and intervening 4.5 mg twice-daily doses, but many patients cannot tolerate 12 mg of rivastigmine each day. The patch comes in 4.6 mg and 9.5 mg strengths, with the higher dose being used after one month on 4.6 mg. Although the patches avoid peak and trough plasma levels and are associated with fewer gastrointestinal side effects than oral rivastigmine, some patients develop skin reactions which may render long-term patch use impossible.

In studies of people with AD, cholinesterase inhibitors produce subtle improvements in cognition and function. Between 30 and 60 minutes of supervisory carer time may be saved each day, MMSE scores may rise by a point or two and the patient may be more alert. An apparent slowing in decline is often seen, equivalent to reversing 3–18 months of deterioration. When the extent of any benefit is unclear, a trial off the drug for two to four weeks may indicate (through noticeable worsening of function or behaviour) that the treatment was giving some benefit, in which case it should be restarted. Cessation of a cholinesterase inhibitor in an AD patient who showed an initial drug response should be considered when the patient is severely impaired and no longer mobile, or in a stage where palliative care is indicated. Patients should always be reviewed frequently when cholinesterase inhibitors are ceased, as even quite impaired patients often seem worse when the drug is stopped and improve when it is restarted.

DLB patients and some with Parkinson's Disease Dementia (PDD) sometimes show startling improvement when treated with a cholinesterase inhibitor, although far less trial evidence is available to support their use for these indications. Improvements seen may include a diminution of psychiatric symptoms as well as improvement in cognition, and may reflect the fact that the reticular activating system is cholinergically driven and tends to be dysfunctional in both DLB and PDD.

Memantine

Memantine is an *N*-methyl-D-aspartate (NMDA) receptor antagonist which regulates calcium flux across membranes and may protect against neuronal death. Trials suggest that it has modest efficacy in retarding the progression of moderate to severe AD and may be helpful in mild AD and some forms of VaD. It is usually well tolerated and the standard dose is 10 mg twice daily, although a 20 mg preparation given once per day is also available now. Its use may be considered in AD patients who do not tolerate a cholinesterase inhibitor or concomitantly with a cholinesterase inhibitor when AD patients are deteriorating despite the prescription of a cholinesterase inhibitor drug. Memantine is subsidized in fewer places than are the cholinesterase inhibitor drugs, and in some countries it is not possible to have both types of drug subsidized simultaneously for the same patient.

Drug treatment of VaD

It is usual to treat hypertension and to use aspirin as secondary prophylaxis in people with VaD, but evidence of efficacy for retarding cognitive deterioration is scant. Where atrial fibrillation is present, anti-arrhythmics and warfarin may be considered for use. Some trial evidence supports the use of cholinesterase inhibitors and/or memantine in patients with VaD, although they do not seem to be helpful when only one large infarct is present.

Other drugs

The use of psychotropic drugs in people with dementia will be addressed in Chapter 5.

A number of putative disease-modifying treatments for AD are under development. Most focus on one or more elements of the amyloid cascade. While it is quite likely that one or more disease-modifying treatments for AD will become available before 2020, the greatest potential for such treatments may be in the prophylactic treatment of healthy people at high risk of developing AD in future.

Social management

Referral to a local Alzheimer association or society for education and advice should be offered to all newly diagnosed dementia patients and their carers. Driving should be assessed if the person with dementia wants to keep driving. If the patient is competent to cede enduring power of attorney and make any changes to an existing Will or draft a new one, these things should be done soon after diagnosis.

A wide variety of community supports such as day centres, in-home respite, home help, bathing attendants, visiting nurses and carer support groups is available in most developed countries and their use should be discussed with patients and families at the start of the illness and at routine follow-up visits thereafter.

The utilization of residential care for people with dementia varies markedly around the globe. The best care homes have activity programmes for residents and sufficient trained staff to attend to their needs, including psychological as well as physical needs. There is growing interest in psychiatric consultation to residential care facilities by multi disciplinary teams who work closely with GPs, nurses and allied health staff in such settings.

Carer support

Family carers of dementia patients experience much higher levels of burden, stress and distress than age-matched members of the general population. Considerable research evidence now indicates that many of the adverse consequences of caring can be prevented or minimized by education, support and intervention, especially when this assistance commences at an early stage of the dementia. Therefore, in dementia care the 'real' patient is comprised of the dyad of the person with dementia and their main carer. Timely medical, psychological and practical support matched to the needs of the patient and their carer should be planned and implemented at an early stage to anticipate, forestall and manage the inevitable stresses and strains that accompany caring for a person with dementia. In most countries contact with the local Alzheimer association offers an ideal starting point for access to education, information and support to carers.

Outcome

It has been said that life is a sexually transmitted fatal disease. People with dementia do die eventually, just like the rest of us. They die excessively in accidents and of pneumonia. Quality of life in mild and even moderately demented patients is often surprisingly good, but suffering and distress are more common in the later stages of the syndrome. In advanced dementia the utility of medical treatment of incident illnesses needs to be balanced against the likelihood of producing any meaningful improvement in quality of life and the long-term prognosis of the illness. Getting clear information about the patient's views on life-prolonging treatments at an early stage of the dementia can inform practice when dementia is advanced and families should be closely involved in decisions about end of life care.

Conclusion

The last 30 years have seen remarkable advances in our understanding of dementia and our management of the syndrome. People with dementia and their carers should have the right to receive a standard of care informed by the knowledge accumulated over this time, and as a consequence the experience of dementia should be far better for current and future generations than for past ones. With the current rapid and sustained increase in biological, clinical and social research into the dementias, a very bright light can at last be seen shining at the end of the dementia tunnel.

FURTHER READING

Articles

Almeida, O., Flicker, L. and Lautenschlager, N. L. (Guest editors). (2005). Uncommon dementias. *International Psychogeriatrics*, **17** (Suppl. 1).
Very comprehensive and detailed coverage of the less common but nevertheless important types of dementia, including early-onset dementias.

Ames, D., Kaduskiewicz, H., van den Bussche, H., Zimmerman, T., Birks, J. and Ashby, D. (2008). For debate: is the evidence for the efficacy of cholinesterase inhibitors in the symptomatic treatment of Alzheimer's disease convincing or not? *International Psychogeriatrics*, **20**, 259–292.
The final word(s) on the controversy about the utility of cholinesterase inhibitors to treat AD?

Clarfield, A. M. (2003). The decreasing prevalence of reversible dementias: an updated meta-analysis. *Archives of Internal Medicine*, **163**, 2219–2229.
An excellent summary of the evidence in relation to the nature and prevalence of so-called reversible dementias.

Ritchie, C. W., Ames, D., Clayton, T. and Lai, R. (2004). Meta-analysis of randomized trials of the efficacy and safety of donepezil, galantamine and rivastigmine for the treatment of Alzheimer's disease. *American Journal of Geriatric Psychiatry*, **12**, 358–369.
A good overview of the evidence for the utility of the class of drugs most often used to treat AD.

Books

Ames, D., Burns, A., and O'Brien, J. T. (Eds). 2010. *Dementia,* 4th edition. London: Hodder Arnold.
An encyclopaedic 700-page compilation of information about all aspects of dementia.

Burns, A. and Waldemar, G. (2009). *Alzheimer's Disease.* Oxford: Oxford University Press.
A brief but comprehensive overview of the commonest form of dementia.

Ritchie, C., Ames, D., Masters, C., and Cummings, J. (Eds.) (2007). *Therapeutic Strategies in Dementia.* Oxford: Clinical Publishing.
A detailed overview of all treatment and management options in dementia including cognitive enhancing agents.

5

Behavioural and psychological symptoms of dementia

Introduction

Although the cognitive aspects of dementia have attracted great attention from researchers, in addition to her cognitive difficulties, Alzheimer's original patient, Augusta D, exhibited agitation, paranoid delusions and mood symptoms which were the main reasons for her admission to hospital, and it is far more common for behavioural symptoms rather than cognitive decline to prompt entry to long-term care.

Systematic study of what variously have been termed the non-cognitive, neuropsychiatric behavioural and psychological, or behavioural and psychiatric symptoms of dementia dates back only to the mid-1980s, and it is only since that time that robust scales for rating these phenomena have emerged. Consequently descriptive and intervention studies have proliferated over the last two decades.

The term 'Behavioural and Psychological Symptoms of Dementia (BPSD)' arose from a consensus conference organised by the International Psychogeriatric Association (IPA). The varied and diffuse nature of the symptoms grouped under this heading (see Table 5.1) limits the utility of the term, but its promulgation has done much to draw attention to this heterogeneous and important collection of phenomena.

Specific symptoms

Table 5.1 lists common BPSD symptoms exhibited by people with dementia. Over 60% of elderly people with dementia living in the community are reported by relatives to exhibit one or more of these symptoms at any given time, and in half of these cases the symptom is at least of moderate intensity, while over 90% of people with dementia will exhibit at least one BPSD that needs specific management at some point in the course of their illness. However, it is important to note that while it is common for individuals with dementia to exhibit such symptoms, these phenomena tend to wax and wane over time and certain symptoms are characteristic of certain stages of the dementia syndrome, and some symptoms (e.g. visual hallucinations in dementia with Lewy bodies) are more common in some dementias than in others.

BPSD is an umbrella term. People with dementia who exhibit BPSD have in common the fact that they have a dementia and experience symptoms or

Table 5.1 Behavioural and psychological symptoms of dementia.

Mood symptoms
Depression
Anxiety
Euphoria
Apathy
Psychotic symptoms
Delusions
Hallucinations
Misidentifications
Vegetative disorders
Sleep–wake cycle disturbances
Disorders of motor behaviour
Sexual disinhibition or aggression
Other phenomena
Resistance to care interventions
Unprovoked physical or verbal aggression
Disruptive vocalization (noisy behaviour)

Note: Treatment should be targeted to the relief of specific symptoms.

behaviours which trouble either themselves or those around them. However, the diffuse nature of BPSD implies that every patient needs an individualized assessment and that the management strategy for one type of BPSD symptom usually will be very different to that required for another type or group of symptoms.

Natural history of BPSD

Symptoms of depression and anxiety are common in the premonitory stages of dementia before a diagnosis has been made, as well as in patients with mild dementia. While it is not uncommon for anxiety symptoms to be present at later stages of dementia, depressive symptoms tend to be less common in advanced dementia, although such symptoms are harder to assess in a moderately to severely demented individual in whom assessment of mood by traditional mental state examination may be rendered difficult by comprehensive and expressive language difficulties.

Delusions and hallucinations are uncommon in very mild dementia, but become more common as dementia advances. Misidentifications of formerly familiar people and places can lead to marked agitation as individuals seek to leave their homes to find some former residence or reject individual family members whom they no longer recognize. As is the case with depressive symptoms, patients with very advanced dementia rarely manifest clear-cut hallucinatory or delusional phenomena, but again, eliciting a description of such experiences from a person with severe dementia may be all but impossible.

Perhaps the commonest reason for a psychiatrist to be asked to assess a person with dementia living in residential care is because of resistance to care interventions or aggressive behaviour directed towards other residents or staff. Although such resistive behaviour tends to be due to an inability to comprehend the need for or the nature of care interventions, the progressive loss of physical condition and mobility that accompany the dementia syndrome in its advanced stages often render such aggressive and resistive behaviour less problematic.

Apathy is the commonest BPSD symptom in advanced dementia.

Assessment of the patient with possible BPSD

It is essential to ask both patients and carers (these may be family members or professional staff) about BPSD symptoms whenever a patient with a dementia is assessed for the first time or reviewed in routine follow-up. The emergence of troublesome BPSDs often acts as a trigger for referral of a patient with dementia to psychiatric services.

The usual routine of history (both from patient and key informants), mental state examination (including an examination of cognitive function), physical examination and targeted special investigations should be followed (in females a mid-stream urine specimen will quite often reveal some degree of infection). Among the key questions which need to be addressed are:

- What symptoms are exhibited?
- When, where and in what circumstances are these symptoms manifest?
- Who (if anybody) is troubled by these symptoms and why?
- What management strategies have been tried to date and how effective have they been?

Several instruments have been developed to assess aspects of BPSD. Among the most popular are Cummings' Neuropsychiatric Inventory (NPI) and the Cohen Mansfield Agitation Inventory (CMAI).

It is common for treatable physical conditions to exacerbate or cause certain BPSDs and sometimes drug treatment of these can make the problem worse. For example, severe constipation can lead to distress and agitation, but some antipsychotic or antidepressant medications can cause or worsen constipation. Pain from an arthritic hip or discomfort from a urinary tract infection can also be effectively managed without recourse to powerful psychotropic drugs.

Management principles

The Latin phrase *primum non nocere* (first do no harm) is nowhere more applicable than in the management of individuals with BPSD. Although there is some evidence for the utility of certain psychosocial interventions, and some psychotropic drugs have been subject to reasonably rigorous evaluation, it is still fair to say that most interventions lack a large body of robust evidence to support their use, and that even where that evidence has been collected, some treatments, especially those that involve drugs, carry with them a significant risk of adverse effects, some of which can be disabling or, rarely, fatal. Finally, the protean nature of BPSD means that any 'one size fits all' approach is bound to be ineffective in many cases. It may be a good idea to treat a miserable, weeping patient with appetite reduction and early morning waking with an antidepressant, but the use of an antipsychotic for such an individual on the grounds that these drugs 'have been shown to be helpful in BPSD' may make the situation worse.

In general, once treatable medical causes for BPSD have been eliminated or addressed with appropriate therapies, the standard approach to treatment is to try psychosocial interventions first, followed by a cautious introduction of psychotropic drug monotherapy in cases where there is some evidence of possible efficacy. However, although one would not ordinarily turn immediately to drug therapy, this may be necessary when symptoms are severe or of a specific type (e.g. delusions) that might be expected to respond to specific medication.

Non-pharmacological management

Not long ago, an expert in this field wrote that research into the non-pharmacological management of dementia was characterized by unsupported assertions and unreplicated results. Things have improved since those words were written, but it is true that most outcome data from psychosocial intervention studies are characterized by sub-optimal sample sizes, that some studies employ less than robust outcome measures, and that a number of approaches which show promising potential have not yet been subject to rigorous, replicated, randomized controlled trials.

Six basic approaches to treatment can be characterized:

1. Person- and family-centred approaches emphasize the need to understand the life history and sociocultural background of the person with dementia and their significant others. While the approach has some acknowledged limitations, it seems axiomatic that such information may at least contribute to making some of the patient's behaviours more understandable for staff and may lead to more appropriate management. One example of such an approach is the case of a former wool-classer who spent much of the day disrupting bed coverings and shaking them out, as he would have done with wool fleeces years earlier. When he was given a pile of blankets, a table, and a room to shake them in, and invited to take a break for 'smokoe' once every two hours, staff of the residential facility where he lived found his behaviour to be better contained and easier to deal with.
2. Caring for carers emphasizes the fact that carers have needs for self-fulfilment and activity which in most cases are not entirely fulfilled by caring for their demented relative, even where this is not explicitly admitted or acknowledged. A number of evidence-based approaches have focused on caring for carers. Support such as in-home respite or carer support groups may help to address some of these needs and make it easier for a tired, frustrated carer to continue the caring role.
3. One randomized controlled trial (RCT) has indicated that nurse practitioners using a collaborative care model may offer effective help to manage BPSD.
4. Community outreach, again focused on the provision of assistance, and advice provided by nurses also has supportive evidence from a single RCT.

5. The utilization of implicit memory has been the subject of one nurse-centred RCT and again shows promise.
6. Finally, the use of non-contingent positive regard (be nice to people and they are more likely to be nice to you) has anecdotal and some trial evidence for its utility. Certainly there is no published evidence to indicate that being unpleasant to people with dementia does anyone any good!

These six approaches can be boiled down to three major avenues of assistance. One is to utilize behaviour management techniques to diminish the frequency of undesirable behaviours through positive reinforcement of desirable ones. The second is to train and empower both family and professional carers through education, and thereby to enhance their management skills, and thus to diminish the negative consequences (burden, stress, anxiety, depression) of caring. A third approach is the utilization of specific interventions for specific behaviours. The simulated presence of a significant other (often through tape recording of voice) is reported to be effective in diminishing both physical and verbal agitation. The use of music, individually matched to the past preferences of the individual receiving therapy, appears helpful in diminishing physical agitation. Structured physical activity improves competence in activities of daily living, but does not diminish the frequency or intensity of behaviours of concern. Finally, aromatherapy, while popular, has only modest evidence to support its use in the amelioration of BPSD (lavender oil is the most promising agent assessed to date).

Pharmacological management

Table 5.2 lists a large number of drug treatments, all of which have but two things in common. First, all of these drugs have at some time been used or advocated for use in treating or controlling certain BPSD. Second, none of these drugs was developed for the specific purpose of treating individuals with dementia for disturbed behaviour or psychological symptoms. Therefore, it is not surprising that these treatments do not always 'work' when given to behaviourally disturbed or psychologically distressed individuals affected by dementia.

Antipsychotic drugs

Reasonable evidence exists to suggest that some novel antipsychotic drugs, particularly low-dose risperidone in doses between 0.5 mg and 2 mg daily (use of risperidone for this purpose has been better studied than is the case for any other drug), may have modest efficacy in ameliorating psychosis, aggression, and agitation. The effect is not mediated solely by the induction of somnolence, and while the evidence is best for risperidone, there are some positive indications for the use of olanzapine, and one trial supports the possible use of aripiprazole for this indication. No other novel antipsychotic has evidence of efficacy in this regard. Evidence for the older classical antipsychotic drugs such as haloperidol is weaker, as most of the few, small trials of these drugs took place before the development of modern instruments for the evaluation of efficacy.

Table 5.2 Drugs that have been used or advocated for the treatment of BPSD – few have clear efficacy and many have significant adverse effects.

Novel antipsychotics
Classical antipsychotics
Antidepressants
Benzodiazepines
Lithium
Anticonvulsants (valproate, carbemazepine)
Barbiturates
Cholinesterase inhibitors
Oestrogen
Cyproterone acetate

Unfortunately, there is strong evidence that classical antipsychotics commonly cause troublesome extra-pyramidal side effects in people with dementia, that they may exacerbate Parkinsonism and may occasionally be associated with fatal adverse events when used to treat people with DLB. Use of the novel antipsychotics risperidone and olanzapine in people with dementia is associated with threefold increase in the risk of (both serious and non-serious) cerebrovascular adverse events (CVAEs), and there is some evidence to suggest that this risk is at least as high, if not higher, when classical antipsychotics are used for the same indication. To date, the mechanism by which the risk of such CVAEs is raised remains obscure, but effects on blood pressure and coagulability do not seem to explain the risk. Individuals with poorly controlled cardiac arrhythmias, hypertension, diabetes and previous stroke were very much over-represented in the group experiencing CVAEs in trials, and it is likely that the risk will be substantially lower in dementia patients who do not exhibit these risk factors.

Antidepressants

Reasonably good-quality evidence has been obtained in studies which randomized a modest number of subjects to suggest that both sertraline and citalopram may be helpful to ameliorate the depressive syndromes sometimes seen in dementia. Although the use of SSRI antidepressants can be associated with agitation, most dementia patients tolerate the newer antidepressants quite well. Tricyclic antidepressants are likely to produce anticholinergic side effects and should not be used to treat depression (or anything else) in most people with dementia, as their central cholinergic systems are likely to be malfunctioning already, without the addition of an anticholinergic drug.

Other psychotropic drugs

Cholinesterase inhibitors appear to have a detectable but weak effect in delaying the emergence of BPSD in individuals with AD who start treatment when mildly demented. Any evidence that such drugs are effective in treating prevalent agitation or other BPSD symptoms in more severely demented individuals is lacking or at best extremely weak. In other words, early treatment with these drugs may help retard the emergence of BPSD in addition to any other benefits on cognition, activity, or carer time required for supervision and assistance, but they are not first choice therapy for any element of BPSD in more advanced AD. In DLB there is evidence from one RCT that rivastigmine may have significant benefit in ameliorating hallucinations, delusions and agitation.

Despite advocacy for their use made on the basis of early small studies, most trials of anticonvulsants in the management of BPSD (these trials have focused upon the use of sodium valproate and carbamazepine, but single negative trials of gabapentin, lamotrigine and topiramate also have been reported) have been negative, and a recent, thorough review of the literature concluded that there was no convincing basis upon which to advocate their routine use.

In summary, the antidepressants sertraline and citalopram should be first choice for therapeutic use in depressed people with dementia. Where aggression or psychosis are prominent, low-dose risperidone (0.5–2 mg daily) is the drug of choice, with olanzapine (2.5–10 mg daily) as second line therapy if extra-pyramidal side effects prove problematic. Patients' relatives should be informed of the increased risk of CVAE associated with such therapy. Excluding individuals at high risk of stroke may diminish the incidence of such events. Cholinesterase inhibitors may delay the emergence of BPSD in some people with AD, but there is little evidence for the efficacy of any other psychotropic drugs in managing BPSD.

Conclusions

In no area of old age psychiatry is the need for more research on effective safe therapies which show reasonable efficacy more pressing than in the area of BPSD. Current best practice should involve the thorough assessment of individuals with dementia who exhibit aggressive or distressing behaviours or dysphoric psychological symptoms, the optimal management of any underlying or co-morbid medical problems, evaluation and manipulation of environmental precipitants, education of both professional and family carers, the use of some specific behavioural interventions in some cases, and the cautious use of antidepressants or novel antipsychotics where specifically indicated for individual symptoms of moderate or greater severity.

FURTHER READING

Articles

Ames, D., Ballard, C., Cream, J., Shah, A., Suh, G-H. and McKeith, I. (2005). For debate: should novel antipsychotics ever be used to treat the behavioral and psychological symptoms of dementia (BPSD)? *International Psychogeriatrics*, **17**, 3–29.
This article summarizes the pros and cons of using antipsychotics to treat BPSD.

Brodaty, H. *et al.* (2003). A randomized placebo controlled trial of Risperidone for the treatment of agitation and psychosis of dementia. *Journal of Clinical Psychiatry,* **64**, 134–143.
A good example of a well-conducted drug trial, this paper illustrates the challenges of conducting such studies as well as highlighting both beneficial and adverse effects of therapy.

Cohen Mansfield, J., *et al.* (1989). A description of agitation in a nursing home. *Journal of Gerontology,* **44**, M77–M84.
This paper contains a description of the Cohen Mansfield Agitation Inventory, one of the most widely used and useful scales in the assessment of BPSD.

Cummings, J. L. *et al.* (1994). The Neuropsychiatric Inventory: comprehensive assessment of psychopathology in dementia. *Neurology,* **44**, 2308–2314.
Konovalov, S., Murali, S. and Tampi, R. R. (2008). Anticonvulsants for the treatment of behavioral and psychological symptoms of dementia: a literature review. *International Psychogeriatrics,* **20**, 293–308.
This review concludes that there is little evidence to support the use of anticonvulsants to treat BPSD.

O'Connor, D., Ames, D., Gardner, B. and King, M. (2009). Psychosocial treatments of behavior symptoms in dementia: a systematic review of reports meeting quality standards. *International Psychogeriatrics,* **21**, 225–240.
O'Connor, D., Ames, D., Gardner, B. and King, M. (2009). Psychosocial treatments of psychological symptoms in dementia: a systematic review of reports meeting quality standards. *International Psychogeriatrics,* **21**, 241–251.
These two review articles deal with the psychosocial management of BPSD and are the most up to date and comprehensive of their type.

Books

Ames, D., Burns, A., and O'Brien, J. T. (2010). *Dementia,* 4th edition. London: Hodder Arnold.
This comprehensive textbook covers virtually all aspects of dementia and has good chapters on the assessment and management of BPSD, including psychosocial and pharmacological approaches.

Dowden, J. *et al.* (2008). *Therapeutic Guidelines Psychotropic Version 6.* Melbourne: Therapeutic Guidelines Ltd.
An excellent guide to the utilization of psychopharmacological strategies in all forms of mental illness including dementia.

Ritchie, C., Ames, D., Masters, C., and Cummings, J. (2007). *Therapeutic Strategies in Dementia.* Oxford: Clinical Publishing.
A thorough review of all aspects of dementia treatment including BPSD.

6

Delirium

Introduction

Delirium in old age is common, clinically important, costly, and potentially preventable. It is the most frequent complication following hospital admission in this age group, and in many instances it is due to a failure of care. Health professionals sometimes lack the necessary knowledge, skills and attitudes to assess, manage and prevent delirium in the modern high-technology, fast-throughput hospital environment, and the consequence is adverse outcomes for patients and a huge waste of resources for services. There is evidence that interventions can reduce the incidence of hospital-acquired delirium, and limit its impact should it occur.

Clinical features

Delirium was one of the first mental disorders to be identified; recognizable descriptions of transient derangements of mental functioning due to illness, injury and intoxication can be found in the ancient Greek Hippocratic texts. The subsequent history of the concept is complex and confusing, but the following have consistently been recognized as core features: disturbance of consciousness, disturbance of thinking (cognition), rapid onset, fluctuating course, and evidence of some external cause. It is an acute disorder, and usually resolves with treatment of the underlying causes, but the longer-term outcomes for older patients are often poor, as we shall see.

There are no diagnostic tests for delirium, and making the diagnosis depends upon a careful assessment of its clinical characteristics. The key differential diagnoses are other causes of cognitive impairment, notably dementia in elderly patients, but this distinction is complicated by the fact that dementia is an important risk factor for delirium, and often underlies it. A history of rapid onset (within days) and fluctuating course of cognitive impairment is strongly indicative of a delirium, but the patient will usually not be in a position to describe this, and a collaborative history from family, care staff or nursing records is essential. In some instances, the onset of a delirium can be more insidious, for example the slow accumulation of drugs, but even here the development is over weeks rather than the months or years that are more typical for a dementia.

Delirium is not an all-or-nothing phenomenon, and a full-blown episode meeting formal diagnostic criteria is usually preceded by a prodromal phase as the disorder develops. In some cases, the delirium may resolve before the full syndrome develops, and never achieve diagnostic status. In this prodromal phase, the patient may be able to cooperate with formal mental state assessment, and will describe feeling muddled and unable to concentrate. Perceptions of time and space are distorted, and it takes effort to keep a grip on reality. The sleep–wake cycle is often disturbed in the early stages with sleep during the day and alertness at night, and patients may feel either irritable or lethargic. As the delirium develops, the disturbance of consciousness leads to progressively reduced awareness of the external environment, and reduction of the ability to focus, sustain and shift attention; it is probably this attentional deficit that quickly alerts more experienced clinicians to the possibility of the diagnosis. Cognitive impairments in delirium include disorientation in time and place, memory deficits and language disturbances. Sensory perception, both visual and auditory, may also be disturbed, resulting in misinterpretations, illusions and hallucinations. Patients interviewed about their experiences following an episode of delirium describe an awareness of their confused state, and how they struggle to regain control and understanding of their situation. The acute mental disturbances of delirium are often very frightening and distressing for patients, who may respond with agitated and aggressive behaviour. If the delirium is severe, or if there is significant accompanying dementia, formal mental state assessment may not be possible, and the delirium will need to be inferred from the effects it has on behaviour and other aspects of functioning, such as mobility, continence and activities of daily living.

One of the diagnostic problems with delirium is that it can manifest itself in a hyperactive form, in a hypoactive form, or in a combination or alteration between these states. The exemplar for the hyperactive form of delirium is the acute alcohol withdrawal state known as delirium tremens: the patient is aroused and irritable, and often angry, fearful and aggressive in response to hallucinations in a range of modalities. There may be autonomic arousal, and neurological symptoms such as tremor and myoclonus. By contrast, in hypoactive delirium there is drowsiness, apparent apathy, and underactivity, with slowing of thought, speech and movement. Hyperactive delirium is more often seen in younger adults, and perhaps for this reason has tended to dominate the historical descriptions that underpin modern perceptions of and criteria for the disorder. It is clinically conspicuous, and its detection and diagnosis is relatively straightforward. By contrast, the hypoactive delirium that is seen more often in older adults is much less obvious, particularly if there is a pre-existing dementia. As a result, it is quite common for delirium in an elderly patient to be overlooked by medical and nursing staff – in up to 95% of cases in some studies.

Improving the recognition of delirium is a prerequisite to its effective management, and nurses may be in a better position to do this than doctors, as they are in contact with patients for longer periods of time and can observe fluctuations in the mental state. However, this information needs to be communicated to all members of the clinical team if it is to be useful. Routine, repeated assessment of cognitive function is important, particularly in those patients identified as being at risk of developing delirium. A number of instruments, such as the Confusion Assessment Method (CAM) and the Delirium Rating Scale (DRS) have been developed to assist with the detection and monitoring of delirium, but a simple brief cognitive screen such as the Mini-mental State Examination (MMSE) or clock drawing, while not diagnostic, can also be useful to identify cognitive decline over time, and may be more practical in non-psychiatric settings.

Differential diagnosis

Delirium can mimic most of the organic and functional mental disorders that occur in old age. Like dementia, conditions such as depression, mania and schizophrenia in old age can also predispose to delirium, either through self-neglect or exhaustion, or because of the powerful psychotropic drugs used to treat them, so the possibility of co-morbidity must always be considered. Bear in mind that delirium, like fever or pain, is an important non-specific sign that the patient is physically ill; as a rule, if the diagnosis is in doubt, investigate as if it were a delirium.

Delirium and dementia

In principle, this is an important differential diagnosis to consider, because of the dire consequences of misdiagnosis. In practice, since dementia is the most important vulnerability factor for delirium in elderly patients (see Risk Factors below), co-morbidity is common. Indeed, the appearance of delirium in an apparently cognitively intact elderly individual should prompt a careful assessment for the early signs of dementia once the patient has recovered, since this may be the first sign that the patient is becoming vulnerable in this respect. However, there are pitfalls for the unwary. Faced with a delirious patient, clinicians often become impatient if physical recovery is not quickly followed by cognitive recovery, and if the patient remains cognitively impaired for any length of time this may be attributed to dementia and the patient managed accordingly. In fact, delirium can be quite a persistent disorder in old age, so there is a risk that important life-changing interventions, such as admission to a nursing home, may be made while there is still potential for further cognitive and functional improvement. It has recently been suggested that delirium and dementia may in fact be related at a more fundamental pathophysiological level, as different manifestations of various acute and chronic inflammatory processes in the brain (see Neuropathophysiology below).

Delirium and mood disorders

Depression is another important differential diagnosis of delirium in elderly patients, particularly those with dementia. Like delirium, depression in this group can present with cognitive and functional decline, and disturbances in behaviour and sleep. Diurnal variation in mood may be mistaken for the fluctuations of a delirium, although typically, delirious patients are better in the early part of the day, unlike those with depression. Depression tends to develop more slowly, but within the timescale of a sub-acute delirium. A previous history of episodes of either depression or delirium may be helpful, particularly if the clinical features have been documented.

While depression in old age can sometimes resemble hypoactive delirium, mania is often mistaken for hyperactive delirium. If the patient has a long history of bipolar disorder, the differential diagnosis is not usually problematic, but mania can occur for the first time in old age, often in association with organic cerebral pathology. In all cases, co-morbid delirium is quite common, due to exhaustion and self-neglect.

Neuropathophysiology

The pathogenesis of delirium is not well understood, but many of the functional cortical and sub-cortical areas of the brain are involved, particularly the association cortices, the limbic system and the ascending cholinergic and monoaminergic systems. Electroencephalography (EEG) and evoked potentials show diffuse slowing, and single photon emission computed tomography (SPECT) and positron emission tomography (PET) studies show abnormalities across many brain regions. However, despite this extensive neuronal derangement in response to a wide range of toxic, metabolic and traumatic causes, the relatively limited and stereotyped nature of the core clinical syndrome suggests that there may be a final common pathway for delirium.

There is some evidence for both the structural (neuroanatomical) and functional (neurophysiological) aspects of this pathway. Studies of delirium following stroke suggest it is more common after right-sided (non-dominant) lesions, particularly those involving the posterior parietal cortex and thalamus. At the functional level, there is a growing body of evidence that the delirium is the result of an imbalance in cholinergic and dopaminergic neurotransmission (reduced cholinergic/excess dopaminergic). Muscarinic cholinergic neurotransmission is involved in many of the brain functions that are deranged in delirium: cortical arousal, maintenance of EEG fast-wave activity, REM sleep, memory and learning, maintaining attention, and motor activity. It has long been known that anticholinergic drugs are particularly prone to induce delirium, especially in those whose cholinergic function is already compromised, such as patients with Alzheimer's disease. This drug-induced delirium can be reversed with cholinesterase inhibitor drugs, such as physostigmine. Most anticholinergic drugs act as post- synaptic antagonists, although some may influence cholinergic neurotransmission via pre-synaptic receptors, or more indirectly by influencing other modulating neurons. A number of other causes of delirium, such as hypoxia, hyperglycaemia, thiamine deficiency, liver failure and physical damage, also affect cholinergic neurotransmission by reducing acetylcholine (Ach) synthesis; one of the immediate metabolic precursors of Ach is acetyl-co-enzyme A, an important and potentially rate-limiting component of the aerobic citric acid cycle within the cell. In many parts of the brain, there is a reciprocal interaction between the cholinergic and dopaminergic systems, with increased dopamine activity resulting from reduced cholinergic activity, and vice versa. Not surprisingly, therefore, delirium can be caused by dopamine agonist drugs (e.g. levodopa, bupropion). There is a wide range of dopamine receptor subtypes in the brain, all subserving different functions, and it has been suggested that individual differences in the responsiveness of these, or their differential involvement in different delirium aetiologies, may explain why some delirium is hypoactive (D3 predominant) or hyperactive (D1 predominant). It may be that age-associated changes to the cholinergic and dopaminergic systems, such as reductions in receptor density and plasticity, contribute to increased vulnerability to delirium.

While the cholinergic and dopaminergic systems appear to be the most closely involved in the pathophysiology of delirium, others such as the serotonergic and glutamatergic systems are probably also contributory, either by influence upon the cholinergic/dopaminergic neurons, or in their own right. Delirium is associated with states of both serotonergic excess (e.g. drug-induced 'serotonin syndrome') and insufficiency (e.g. alcohol withdrawal). Some conditions, such as hypoxia, give rise to surges of toxic neurotransmitters (e.g. glutamate) that may be deliriogenic.

How do severe systemic illness, infection and trauma act on the brain to produce delirium? These conditions activate the immune system and stimulate the production of cytokines. One of the functions of these small polypeptides is to communicate with the CNS to elicit 'sickness behaviour' (reduced activity, appetite, social interaction, etc.). They also activate the HPA (hypothalamic–pituitary–adrenal) and HPG (hypothalamic–pituitary–gonadal) axes, alter blood–brain barrier permeability, interfere with cerebral neurotransmission, and reduce the activity of neuroprotective cytokines, any or all of which may contribute to delirium in vulnerable individuals. In young adults this cytokine signalling is self-limiting without any lasting consequences, but it has been suggested that conditions such as Alzheimer's disease with a chronic inflammatory component to their pathophysiology may be accelerated by this process, resulting in more rapid cognitive and functional decline. This may account for the evidence of an association between delirium and subsequent cognitive decline in elderly patients.

Epidemiology

There have been many investigations of the prevalence and incidence of delirium in elderly medical and surgical in-patients, with a wide range of rates reported. There are a number of reasons for this variation: different case definitions of delirium, with more or less strict inclusion criteria; different case-finding procedures, from passive methods such as case note review to more active strategies such as patient interview on one or more occasions, which produce a higher yield; and selection bias, including exclusion of more severely ill and high-risk patients. The variability of prevalence and incidence rates is highest in the earlier, less-standardized surveys. More recent studies suggest prevalence rates of 10–20%, and post-admission incidence rates of 5–10%. Some of the variation is probably due to the greater vulnerability of some patient groups; for example, elderly patients following surgery for hip fracture appear to be at particular risk of developing delirium. These figures translate into a significant burden for health services; it has been estimated that in the USA, delirium complicates the hospital admission of over 2.3 million people per year, involving over 17.5 million in-patient days at a cost of over $US4 billion (1994 prices). Delirium in other settings has been studied less extensively. One particularly vulnerable group is the frail elderly population living in nursing homes; some Scandinavian studies have suggested that the prevalence in this setting may be as high as 60%, which raises important questions about the quality of care provided.

Risk factors

At any age, delirium is the consequence of an interaction between intrinsic vulnerability (predisposing causes) and external insults that affect brain functioning (precipitating causes). In childhood, the principal predisposing cause is the incomplete myelination of the central nervous system. In older adults, neurodegenerative disorders such as dementia are the most important predisposing risk factor for delirium, with an associated relative risk of 5.2 (see section on Delirium and dementia earlier in this chapter). Other predisposing vulnerability factors in this age group include impairments in vision and hearing, which approximately double the risk of developing delirium if present. Physical illness factors that increase the risk of delirium include severity, instability, co-morbidity, functional impairment, malnutrition and dehydration. It is not clear to what extent age itself is a risk factor for delirium, independent of age-associated conditions such as dementia and sensory impairment. Age-related changes in receptor populations, drug binding and metabolism may confer increased vulnerability to this particular cause of delirium; for example, hypoalbuminaemia, which increases the amount of free drug in the plasma, has been shown to be predictive of delirium. However, it should be noted that elderly individuals vary considerably in these respects. Male gender, alcohol abuse, and lower educational attainment have also been identified as predisposing factors for delirium in some studies.

Regarding the precipitating factors, any acute physical illness can cause delirium if the patient is sufficiently vulnerable. Among the commonest causes are infections, metabolic disturbances, and conditions that impair oxygen supply to the brain (Table 6.1). Medication is the other common precipitating cause of delirium in elderly patients; again, any drug has the potential to cause delirium, but

Table 6.1 Factors precipitating delirium.

Medication (prescribed)
Medication (over-the-counter)
Medication (alcohol and illicit drugs)
Infection
Cerebral hypoxia (heart failure, myocardial infarct, stroke, etc.)
Metabolic causes
A combination of the above
Something else

Adapted from Rockwood, K. and MacKnight, C. (2001). *Understanding Dementia: A Primer of Diagnosis and Management*. Halifax, Nova Scotia: PottersWeld Press.

psychotropic agents, narcotic analgesics, dopamine agonists and drugs with anticholinergic properties have the greatest potential in this respect. Many of the drugs commonly prescribed to elderly patients, such as prednisolone, cimetidine and digoxin, have some degree of anticholinergic activity, and it may be the cumulative effect that is important. In more severely demented individuals, urinary retention, faecal impaction and pain may be sufficient to precipitate a delirium, although the mechanisms involved are unclear. Similarly, psychological and environmental disruptions, such as relocation, sleep deprivation, sensory deprivation and bereavement can contribute to or cause delirium in those who are vulnerable.

The experience of surgery provides the elderly patient with many opportunities for developing delirium, including per:-operative hypovolaemia and hypothermia, exposure to psychoactive medication (pre-meds, anaesthetics, analgesics), and post-operative sepsis, immobility, sensory deprivation. In fact, modern, minimally invasive techniques combined – crucially – with the ability to select 'good-risk' patients means that observed rates of delirium in elective surgical populations are quite low. They are much higher in 'poor-risk' groups where surgery is unavoidable, such as hip-fracture patients.

Several factors related to the process of care have been shown to increase the risk of developing delirium in hospital, both as predisposing and precipitating causes. These include the number of procedures undergone by the patient, bladder catheterization, polypharmacy, use of physical restraints, and malnutrition. Furthermore, most hospital environments and procedures are not designed with cognitively impaired patients in mind, and probably contribute to the development of delirium. These predisposing and precipitating risk factors are highly inter-related and multiplicative in their effect, and a number of predictive models have been developed in an attempt to identify those patients at particular risk of developing delirium during their hospital stay.

Course and prognosis

Although usually regarded as a transient disorder, delirium can be prolonged or recurrent in about one-third of elderly patients in hospital; disorientation and memory impairment appear to be particularly slow to recover. Rates of cognitive recovery at discharge from hospital range between 40 and 70%. Some groups, such as those admitted to hospital from nursing homes, appear to have a particularly poor outcome in this respect. Patients who have been delirious are at increased risk of developing dementia subsequently. This may be because those in the very early, preclinical, stages of dementia are more vulnerable to delirium; alternatively, delirium may have persistent neurotoxic effects on the brain. If delirium is shown to contribute to the development of dementia, this will further emphasize the need for primary prevention (see below).

Delirium is associated with significant physical ill-health or intoxication, so it is not surprising that it is associated with a number of adverse outcomes, such as increased mortality and morbidity, increased length of hospital stay, increased dependency and short- and long-term functional decline, and institutionalization following discharge. However, delirium also impedes the processes of diagnosis, management and rehabilitation, and increases the risk of developing other hospital-acquired complications; hypoactive patients may develop pressure sores and chest and urinary tract infections, and hypoactive patients are at risk from hip fracture following falls. Consequently, there is a significant independent association between delirium and the various categories of adverse outcome that have been studied, which underlines the importance of prompt and effective management of the condition, and prevention where possible.

Management

The evidence base for effective management strategies in delirium is still very limited. Clinical reviews and practice guidelines identify four key components to the effective management of delirium in the elderly patient: address the underlying causes; maintain behavioural control; prevent common complications; and rehabilitation.

Address the underlying causes

Effective diagnostic assessment of delirium is the starting point for its management. This should focus on the commonest causes: medications, infections, metabolic disorders, and conditions causing impaired oxygenation of the CNS (e.g. anaemia, congestive cardiac failure, chronic obstructive pulmonary disease). Any newly started, increased, or recently discontinued medications should be considered, as should the possibility of adverse drug interactions. Remember that alcohol is also a drug. Infections in elderly patients are not always obvious, and delirium may be the presenting feature of a chest infection, cellulitis, or a urinary tract infection. Dehydration is a common cause of metabolic disruption leading to delirium, particularly in vulnerable groups such as nursing home populations. Other factors that commonly cause or contribute to delirium, such as sensory impairment, constipation and urinary retention, and pain, should also be identified. It should be borne in mind that a simple cause-and-effect model for delirium in old age is usually inappropriate; any individual case is likely to be the consequence of a number of predisposing and precipitating factors acting together, and all of these need to be addressed in the management. Disruptive and invasive investigations, such as MRI scans or lumbar puncture, are not necessary unless clearly indicated by the clinical history, or if the initial search for common causes is negative.

There are as yet no drugs available that will reverse delirium, although cholinesterase inhibitors are attracting interest in this regard. Delirium secondary to alcohol or sedative withdrawal may be treated with a tapering course of a benzodiazepine such as oxazepam or lorazepam.

Maintain behavioural control

Disturbed behaviour is very poorly tolerated in modern in-patient units, and quickly leads to demands for some form of sedation. However, as with disturbed behaviour in dementia, it is important to consider why the patient is distressed, and address the underlying cause wherever possible. In the case of delirium, this is usually because the patient is unable to make sense of what they perceive as an alien and hostile environment. The reassuring presence of family members can be very helpful, as can the provision of consistent nursing staff. All interactions with the patient should be calm, non-confrontational and orienting, and interventions should be carefully explained in a step-by-step way that the patient can understand. Modifications of hospital environment and routines, including use of non-pharmacological sleep protocols, are effective in restoring normal sleep–wake cycles, but are labour-intensive and hard to achieve in most current hospital systems.

Sometimes chemical or physical restraint may be necessary, to protect the patient or others, but if they are not used with care, they may make the situation worse. Unsupervised physical restraint increases the risk of injury and falls, and excessive or inappropriate psychotropic medication may deepen and prolong the delirium. The limited evidence base in this area favours the use of high-potency antipsychotic drugs such as haloperidol; they are probably most effective when the disturbed behaviour is secondary to psychotic symptoms, such as hallucinations. Initially, haloperidol should be prescribed at a low dose (0.5–1 mg), with frequent review to titrate changes in the dose against response; the aim should be to give the lowest effective dose for the shortest possible time. There is interest in the use of atypical antipsychotic drugs such as risperidone and olanzapine in the management of delirium, but it is not yet clear what advantages they may offer. They may have a role in patients with Parkinson's disease or dementia with Lewy bodies (DLB), where haloperidol should not be used. An alternative would be a benzodiazepine such as lorazepam.

Prevent common complications

Once the underlying causes of the delirium have been corrected, it may take some considerable time for an elderly patient to regain their previous level of functioning, and they will be vulnerable to a wide range of complications that may lead to enduring functional impairment and even death. A crucial aspect of delirium management is to prevent and manage these complications, the commonest of which are: urinary incontinence, immobility, falls, pressure sores, sleep disruption, dehydration and malnutrition. Patients should have a programme of regular toileting (*not* an indwelling catheter), supervised and structured mobilization and physiotherapy, a non-pharmacological sleep hygiene programme, and assistance with feeding, and careful monitoring of food and fluid intake.

Rehabilitation

As the patient recovers, the focus of management shifts to a programme of rehabilitation aimed at a return to the pre morbid state of functioning. The level of basic activities of daily living (ADL) capacity should be assessed regularly, and the patient encouraged to do what they can for themselves wherever possible. The patient's immediate environment should be made as non-threatening and orienting as possible, with regular routines and reminders about the date, time, and place. It is important to involve family members in this process: they are an important source of information about pre morbid functioning; they can contribute to bedside care and support; they have access to familiar and orienting materials, such as photographs; they will have concerns about the cause and the prognosis that will need to be addressed; and they will be heavily involved in the supervision and after-care of the patient once they have been discharged from hospital. Delirium is often recurrent, and the family should be advised to be alert for the early signs of this. There is very little evidence about the effect of post-discharge rehabilitation and support; one study suggests that a relatively modest package of case management and rehabilitation can significantly reduce the use of long-term institutional care. Delirium may be a useful marker of vulnerability in elderly in-patients, and of the need for more intensive community after-care than is usually provided for this population.

Prevention

The evidence base is rather better so far as the prevention of delirium is concerned. An understanding of the multiple risk factors for delirium in hospital settings has led to the development of predictive models, and the evaluation of interventions designed to reduce its incidence. In the Yale–New Haven Study, the intervention consisted of a series of management protocols for cognitive impairment, sleep deprivation, immobility, visual impairment, hearing impairment and dehydration. These were carried out by a trained multidisciplinary team supported by volunteers. When compared to care-as-usual, there was a 40% reduction in the incidence of delirium in the intervention group, with patients at intermediate levels of risk obtaining the greatest benefit. Based on the findings of this study, this programme has been successfully established in three medical units within a hospital, and it appears to be cost-effective.

Studies of geriatric consultation services to general medical and surgical units have produced mixed results; a key factor appears to be the extent to which the recommendations are adhered to by medical and nursing staff.

There is probably more scope for preventing delirium in surgical patients, since the immediate cause is usually planned, and there is time for preparing and optimizing the patient. A range of interventions have been shown to be modestly effective in reducing the incidence of delirium in this population, including pre-operative chest physiotherapy, explanation, support and anxiety management; peri-operative maintenance of blood pressure and oxygen tension; and post-operative pain management, including patient-controlled analgesia.

A common theme across many intervention strategies is the need to educate health professionals in contact with patients about the importance of delirium, its complications, and how to identify and manage it effectively. Occasional and ad-hoc training activities are unlikely to be effective on their own; delirium needs to form part of all medical and nursing school curricula, with clearly defined learning aims and outcomes. If training can be linked to formal ward-based delirium prevention programmes, so much the better.

Conclusion

Delirium may be regarded as a marker of the quality of hospital care, in terms of: physical design, organization and management, the awareness and training of medical and nursing staff in the recognition and effective management of the problem, and links with community support services. Given the mean age of most medical and surgical in-patient populations in developed societies, there is an urgent need to develop hospital environments, systems of care and clinical teams that are equipped to meet their needs. Achieving this alongside the onward march of medical technology will not be easy; demonstrable cost-effectiveness is probably the key.

FURTHER READING

Articles

Brown, T. M. and Boyle, M. F. (2002). Delirium. *BMJ*, **325**, 644–647.
Clear, readable overview from the UK.

Cole, M. (2004). Delirium in elderly patients. *American Journal of Psychiatry*, **12**, 7–21.
Another good overview, this time from a North American perspective.

Inouye, S. K., Schlesinger, M. J. and Lydon, T. J. (1999). Delirium: a symptom of how hospital care is failing older persons and a window to improve quality of hospital care. *American Journal of Medicine*, **106**, 563–573.
This article, whose first author has done as much as anyone to bring the challenge of delirium to clinical attention, is as pertinent now as when it was published.

Meagher, D. J. (2001). Delirium: optimising management. *BMJ*, **322**, 144–149.
Sensible, practical management advice.

Book

Lindesay, J., Rockwood, K., and Macdonald, A. J. D. (2002). *Delirium in Old Age*. Oxford: Oxford University Press.
A comprehensive and useful overview of the topic.

7

Mood disorders in late life

A. DEPRESSION

Introduction

The ubiquity of losses in old age has sometimes invited the conclusion that depression is an inevitable consequence of living into late life. However, evidence does not support this hypothesis and, hence, one must be vigilant about dismissing depressive symptoms in older adults as inevitable. The clinical implication is that those patients with persistent depressive symptoms as defined below must be taken seriously and properly assessed and managed.

Nosology and classification

The diagnosis of depression is defined in contemporary psychiatry by the classification systems of the American Psychiatric Association (DSM-IV) as well as the International Classification of Diseases (ICD-10). Tables 7.1 and 7.2 outline the definitions for both DSM-IV and ICD-10 of major depression, milder depression, and dysthymia.

Medical and neurologic co-morbidity

Compared to a mixed-aged population, older adults experience a high level of co-morbidity of medical diseases as well as cognitive disorders, including dementias and other forms of mild cognitive impairment. These two features make depression, particularly late-onset depression, a challenge to diagnose and treat.

Cognitive impairment, dementia and the phenomenology of depression

Notwithstanding the evidence suggesting that late-life depression sometimes may be a prodrome of dementia, there is also a substantial body of evidence to suggest that depression represents an independent risk factor that predisposes to dementia. This is true even when depressive symptoms occur many years prior to

Table 7.1 Classification and diagnosis of geriatric depressive disorders.

Major depressive disorder

A. Five of the following symptoms must be present: depressed mood, diminished interest or loss of pleasure in all or almost all activities, weight loss or gain (more than 5% of body weight), insomnia or hypersomnia, psychomotor agitation or retardation, fatigue, feelings of worthlessness or inappropriate guilt, reduced ability to concentrate, recurrent thoughts of death or suicide.

At least one of the symptoms must be either depressed mood or diminished interest or pleasure. The syndrome should last at least two weeks, lead to distress or functional impairment, and not be a direct effect of substance use, a medication condition, or bereavement.

Note: *Symptoms that are clearly due to a general medical condition are not included, nor are mood-incongruent delusions or hallucinations.*

(1) Depressed mood most of the day, nearly every day, as indicated by either subjective report (e.g. feels sad or empty) or observation made by others (e.g. appears tearful).

(2) Marked diminished interest or pleasure in all, or almost all, activities most of nearly every day (as indicated by either subjective account or observation made by others).

(3) Significant weight loss when not dieting or weight gain (e.g. a change of more than 5% of body weight in a month), or decrease or increase in appetite nearly every day.

(4) Insomnia or hypersomnia nearly every day.

(5) Psychomotor agitation or retardation nearly every day (observable by others, not merely subjective feelings of restlessness or being slowed down).

(6) Fatigue or loss of energy nearly every day.

(7) Feelings of worthlessness or excessive or inappropriate guilt (which may be delusional) nearly every day (not merely self-reproach or guilt about being sick).

(8) Diminished ability to think or concentrate or indecisiveness nearly every day (either by subjective account or as observed by others).

(9) Recurrent thoughts of death (not just fear of dying), recurrent suicidal ideation without a specific plan, or a suicide attempt, or a specific plan for committing suicide.

B. The symptoms do not meet the criteria for a mixed episode.

C. The symptoms cause clinically significant distress or impairment in social, occupational, or other important areas of functioning.

D. The symptoms are due to the direct physiological effects of a substance (e.g. a drug of abuse, a medication) or a general medical condition (e.g. hypothyroidism).

E. The symptoms are not better accounted for by bereavement, i.e. after the loss of a loved one, the symptoms persist for longer than 2 months or are characterized by marked functional impairment, morbid preoccupations with worthlessness, suicidal ideation, psychotic symptoms, or psychomotor retardation

Specifiers can be coded for *severity* (mild, moderate, or severe); *psychosis* (mood-congruent or mood-incongruent delusions or hallucinations); and *remission* (partial or full).

Minor depressive disorder

At least two but fewer than five of the symptoms of major depressive disorder must be present.

The syndrome should last at least two weeks, lead to distress or functional impairment, and not be a direct effect of substance use, a medication condition, or bereavement.

Table 7.1. (*cont.*)

This diagnosis can only be made in patients without a history of major depression, dysthymia, bipolar, or psychotic disorders.

Dysthymic disorder
Sad mood for more days than not, accompanied by another two symptoms of major depressive disorder.
A duration of at least two years is required.
An episode of major depression might not be present during the first two years of the disorder.

Bipolar 1 disorder (most recent episode depressed)
Individuals meet criteria for major depressive disorder and have a history of at least one manic episode or a mixed episode.

Adjustment disorder with depressed mood
Individuals who develop depressed mood, tearfulness, or hopelessness within three months of the occurrence of a stressor.
The syndrome should lead to great distress or disability, and should subside within six months of the removal of the stressor.
Bereavement is not considered a stressor for an adjustment disorder.

Reproduced from Alexopoulos, G. S. (2005). Depression in the elderly. *Lancet,* **365,** 1961–1970, with permission from Elsevier.

Table 7.2 ICD-10 depressive episode.

A. The syndrome of depression must be present for at least two weeks; no history of mania; and not attributable to organic disease or psychoactive substance

Mild depressive episode
B. At least two of the following three symptoms must be present:
  (1) Depressed mood to a degree that is definitely abnormal for the individual, present for most of the day and almost every day, largely uninfluenced by circumstances, and sustained for at least two weeks.
  (2) Loss of interst or pleasure in activities that are normally pleasurable.
  (3) Decreased energy or increased fatiguability.
C. An additional symptom or symptoms from the following (at least four):
  (1) Loss of confidence or self-esteem.
  (2) Unreasonable feelings of self-reproach or excessive and inappropriate guilt.
  (3) Recurrent thoughts of death or suicide, or any suicidal behaviour.
  (4) Complaints or evidence of diminished ability to think or concentrate, such as indecisiveness or vacillation.
  (5) Change in psychomotor activity, with agitation or retardation (either subjective or objective).
  (6) Sleep disturbance of any type.
  (7) Change in appetite (decrease or increase) with corresponding weight change.

Moderate depressive episode
As above, but at least six of the symptoms under section C.

Severe depressive episode
All three from Section B and at least five from Section C (eight symptoms in total).

Severe cases may be further subdivided according to the presence or otherwise of psychosis and/or stupor

the onset of dementia. Indeed, lifetime history of depression represents a significant increase in risk of Alzheimer's disease (AD), independent of family history for dementia. Similarly, there is evidence that a history of depression is a risk factor for vascular dementia as well as AD.

Several studies have noted a prevalence of 30–50% for depressive symptoms in AD (the most common of the dementias – see Chapter 4). This very high prevalence of depressive symptoms has also been noted to be persistent in the course of AD and to occur relatively early in the disease. In an attempt to clarify the natural course and prevalence of depressive symptoms in AD, a recent study followed patients with probable AD for up to 14 years. It was demonstrated that the prevalence of depressive symptoms remained stable at approximately 40% during the first few years of follow-up, but then dropped significantly.

The relationship between cognitive impairment and the phenomenology of depression in older adults has been examined to determine whether patients with greater cognitive impairment were more likely to endorse specific symptoms independent of the level of depression. Overall, cognitive impairment was associated with greater depression severity. Patients with more severe levels of cognitive impairment were more likely to complain of greater social withdrawal. In contrast, symptoms such as lack of initiative and depressed mood were not as affected by level of cognitive impairment and were more sensitive to the level of depression. Apathy, a very common feature of dementia, was found to be distinct from depression and social withdrawal.

DSM-IV includes a category of 'depression due to a general medical condition'. This diagnosis is given when the depressed mood occurs in the context of an already diagnosed medical illness that appears to be associated with depression. However, this aetiological association may be a tenuous assumption. Medical illnesses are common in an elderly depressed cohort. Moreover, depression is often an antecedent or prodromal symptom of medical co-morbidities and thus may be an early sign of disease, including neurologic disease such as dementia. Conversely, depression may in itself be a risk factor for the development of certain medical illnesses, including vascular disease. On the other hand, medical disorders may contribute to the pathophysiology of depression, especially vascular disease as described below.

There is evidence that depressed subjects report significantly greater medical co-morbidity than control subjects who are not depressed. Primarily, this difference relates to the prevalence of cardiovascular illnesses, such as hypertension and atherosclerotic heart disease, but also occurs with gastrointestinal ulcers. Hypertension is more common in those patients with sub-cortical white or grey matter ischaemic lesions.

Other evidence supporting the relationship between vascular disease and depression in late life includes the fact that 25% of older individuals who experience a myocardial infarction or who are undergoing cardiac catheterization also have major depression. Another 25% of those exhibit minor depression. Furthermore, 50% of patients with coronary artery disease and co-morbid major depression have at least one prior episode of major depression. In general, the greater the overall medical burden, the greater the risk of depression seen.

Vascular depression hypothesis

Following the association of high levels of co-morbidity, particularly vascular disease in late-life depression, the vascular depression hypothesis has emerged. This hypothesis is supported by a number of findings including the fact that hyperintensities on MRI scanning appear to be associated with vascular disease. Furthermore, it is late-onset depression that is associated with a greater risk of vascular disease and concomitantly with deep white matter hyperintensities. Consequently, this hypothesis has proposed a number of clinical features that are unique to vascular depression. These include a late age of onset, less depressive ideation, less insight, greater disability for the level of depression, presence of apathy and retardation, and an increased prevalence of cognitive impairment, especially frontal/executive dysfunction. Finally, these patients appear to have a worse prognosis. Nevertheless, the hypothesis is not universally accepted and some counterarguments, such as the apparent lack of increase in the prevalence of depression with age despite a rising prevalence of vascular disease, have been put forward. If it is correct, the vascular depression hypothesis suggests that more aggressive treatment and prevention of cerebrovascular disease might reduce the risk of vascular depression. Specifically, antidepressants that promote ischaemic recovery – that is, enhance dopamine or noradrenaline activity – might be preferentially favoured in vascular depression.

Further to the association of vascular disease in late-onset depression, in 2005, Baldwin and colleagues compared neurological signs in a group of individuals with late-onset depression compared to healthy controls. The late-onset depression group had a higher association with mild neurological abnormalities particularly involving sub-cortical signs. They postulated that both neurodegenerative and vascular changes may be aetiologically related to this increased association with neurologic abnormalities.

Further support for the vascular depression hypothesis comes from another association, namely frontostriatal dysfunction in late-life depression. This type of executive dysfunction is characterized by psychomotor slowing, decreased interest in outside activities and greater than expected impairment in daily function, complicated by lack of insight. Such patients generally show a poor response to antidepressant treatment and have a poor outcome.

The relationship between depression and irreversible cognitive impairment has been addressed in Chapter 3 (on differential diagnosis). However, reversible cognitive impairment at a time of major depression that responds to treatment still leaves these individuals with a significant risk of developing irreversible dementia – approximately 40% within the first three years of follow-up. Thus, the reversible cognitive impairment associated with depression, like delirium, may very well be a harbinger of the later development of irreversible dementia.

Suicide risk

In most epidemiologic studies, the risk of suicide is consistently highest in elderly men. Moreover, the ratio of attempted suicide to completed suicide is lowest in older adults. Perhaps, the most important epidemiological finding is the association of depressive syndromes with suicide in older people. It has been shown that the vast majority (>80%) of older individuals who commit suicide have had a pre-existing major depression. These people have been seen by their family physicians prior to their suicide in a large majority of cases. Unfortunately, the depressive illness is often masked by co-morbid medical conditions. Complaints of somatic symptoms, especially pain, tend to invite treatment of a somatic nature, rather than antidepressant measures which may deal with the real causation. Despite the fact that mood disorders represent the most significant independent risk factor for suicide, somatic illnesses and disability including pain significantly increase that risk, although their effect is probably mediated by depression in a bi-directional fashion. That is, physical illness makes depression worse and depression makes one more likely to be sensitive to physical symptoms.

Elderly people are more likely to use violent means of attempting suicide compared to a younger population. Although suicidal ideation in general decreases with age, the presence of suicidal thoughts does put them at a higher risk compared to younger individuals.

Suicidal ideation must be considered an independent feature of an underlying depression which suggests aggressive treatment of depression even in the face of medical co-morbidity. However, measures to deal with co-morbid pain and treatment of underlying medical disability are still important aspects of the treatment of such individuals.

Pathophysiology

A number of different brain structures have been associated with depression in late life. Alexopoulos and his group have consistently shown evidence of fronto-striatal dysfunction which affects both the presentation and the clinical course of late-life major depression. This, in turn, leads to increased executive dysfunction, psychomotor slowing and may explain the increased feelings of apathy.

The amygdala has also been implicated in depression as it mediates emotions. Vascular disease, such as stroke and sub-cortical ischemic changes, may affect the connections between the amygdala, the medial dorsal thalamic nucleus and the orbital frontal cortex, thus predisposing to depression. Alexopoulos has postulated that the presence of co-morbid and chronic medical illnesses may be associated with increased activity of the amygdala, leading to increasing secretion of cortisol and hence depression. Increased activity of the amygdala in association with inadequate cortical modulation of emotional output may contribute to depression.

Abnormalities of the hippocampus have been associated with both depression and dementia. A number of studies have shown a decreased volume of the hippocampus associated with the first episode of major depression. This may be another factor in the association of dementia and depression.

Epidemiology

It is important to distinguish between the prevalence of depressive symptoms compared to a major depressive episode. Epidemiologic studies show that 10–15% of older adults living in the community report some degree of significant depressive symptomatology. However, only about 0.5–3% of the elderly population in the community are experiencing a major depressive episode at any given time. This is equivalent to an incidence of around 0.15% per year. There is some suggestion that milder forms of depression including minor depression, sub-syndromal depression or dysthymia are somewhat more common in older than in younger adults. However, there is no evidence to show that the incidence or prevalence of major depression increases with advancing age.

The prevalence of late-life depression is higher in medical settings than in the community. Approximately 10% of older adults admitted to hospital exhibit major depression, whereas in primary care 6–9% of older adults have major depression. In nursing homes rates of major depression approximate 12–15%, while depressive *symptoms* occur in the range of 17–35% among people in long-term care. These higher prevalence rates clearly are confounded by medical and neurologic co-morbidity as well as increased disability in that specific population. This is consistent with the robust finding that greater medical burden increases the risk of depression.

Treatment

Before considering specific antidepressant treatments, either pharmacological or psychotherapeutic in nature, a careful assessment of co-morbidities and drug interactions must be undertaken. Given the high prevalence of medical co-morbidity and the polypharmacy associated with depressive illness in older adults, potentially treatable conditions or offending drugs must be identified and addressed.

The limited available evidence suggests that older adults have a similar antidepressant treatment response as mixed-age populations. However, the anticholinergic impact of psychotropics on older adults must be a special consideration, and consequently some experts suggest that the serotonin reuptake inhibitor class (SSRIs) or the serotonin and noradrenergic reuptake inhibitor (SNRIs) are appropriate first-choice medications for an older population. Nevertheless, a number of recent studies suggest that effectiveness and adverse events are not significantly different between tricyclic antidepressants (TCAs) and SSRIs. A recent Cochrane meta-analysis noted that there were difficulties in generalizing results from clinical trials into the general population. However, overall they found the efficacy of SSRIs and TCAs to be very similar. They did find, however, that withdrawal rates from randomized controlled trials were higher for patients taking classical TCAs than those receiving SSRIs. None the less, there did not appear to be a dramatic advantage of newer serotonin reuptake inhibitors compared to the TCAs. The available studies related to older adults are confounded by small numbers, heterogeneity of the samples and a diversity of pharmacological profile of drugs that have often been grouped together for purposes of categorization. Identifying the side-effect profile is compounded by the particular importance in older adults of somatic symptoms of depression as well as the co-morbid medical diseases that may mask the side effects of specific drugs. This is an issue that has received inadequate attention considering the vulnerability to somatic symptoms and side effects of this older population.

While the dictum 'start low, go slow' certainly applies to the treatment of depression in old age, it is also clear that many elderly depressed patients require similar therapeutic doses to younger adults. As long as the antidepressant is well tolerated, one should titrate the dose according to response. A recent review by Alexopoulos has suggested that second-line drugs after SSRIs or SNRIs should include bupropion and mirtazapine. However, in the real world of clinical experience, virtually all classes and all combination therapies (e.g. antidepressant plus lithium, antidepressant plus antipsychotic) may be appropriate for older adults suffering from depression. They should be afforded the same therapeutic armamentarium that younger patients enjoy.

For milder depressions that are initiated by a specific stressor or those with less severity, psychotherapeutic approaches alone or combined with an antidepressant may be a reasonable first step. Available evidence suggests that cognitive behaviour therapy, supportive psychotherapy, problem-solving therapy and interpersonal psychotherapies have all had some efficacy in late-life depression.

Reasons why there appears to be an 'efficacy–effectiveness gap' in an older population have been reviewed (see Mulsant *et al.*, 2003 in the further reading section at the end of this chapter). Efficacy refers to the rate of response and recovery that is observed under ideal research conditions such as a randomized controlled trial. However, whether this response rate can be generalized to the real world is tempered by 'effectiveness', which is the rate of response and recovery that is reported in the 'real world' of clinical care. In older adults, this gap is attributed to the frequent presence of co-morbid medical conditions that may lead to polypharmacy and adverse events as well as a decrease in adherence to medications. For example, cognitive impairment and co-morbid alcoholism are frequent complications encountered when treating older adults with depression. Second, there is evidence to support the targeting of full remission of symptoms, since those with residual symptoms after initial treatment tend to have a much higher rate of relapse. Consequently, the usual treatment measures apply to older adults. These include raising the dose if tolerated for longer periods of time, switching to a different antidepressant class, or adding a second antidepressant or specific augmenting agent. One should always consider including a psychotherapeutic approach to individuals who have had an adequate pharmacological trial but still experience residual symptoms.

Another important initiative to reduce the 'efficacy–effectiveness gap' is by involving carers and family members who will benefit from psychoeducation around the need for ongoing treatment and long-term monitoring. This is more fully described in Chapter 2 (on a assessment). Finally, the management of side effects in a physically and cognitively vulnerable population is especially important. In this regard, the first-choice antidepressant should be one least likely to produce side effects and, hence, the general recommendation of avoiding the anticholinergic TCA agents as first-line treatments.

For refractory depressions in later life, one should consider electroconvulsive therapy (ECT) as an important treatment option, as well as the use of the traditional irreversible monoamine oxidase inhibitors (MAOIs), such as phenelzine or tranylcypromine. Although few clinicians today have much experience or confidence in using these MAOI agents, in a small number of patients they can be effective when all other biological measures have failed. The main complication of ECT when given to old people tends to be transient cognitive impairment, but even quite frail people can tolerate the anaesthetics given for ECT fairly well, and it is the treatment of choice when depression is complicated by delusions, active suicidal behaviour, refusal to eat or drink, or there is a strong history of prior depressive episodes that remitted only after treatment with ECT.

Outcome

Depression at any age tends to be a remitting relapsing disorder. As the length of the depressive episode is the largest factor contributing to poor long-term outcome, initial episodes should be treated energetically as soon as they present. There is some evidence to suggest that recurrent episodes are less likely when prophylactic antidepressant therapy is maintained long-term, but it is likely that the majority of people who experience one episode of late-life depression will have another if they wait long enough. For this reason, it is important that patients and their families are educated to recognize the early symptoms of a depressive relapse and that they are advised to seek review at an early stage if and when such symptoms recur.

Summary

In the management of depression, as in other areas of geriatric psychiatry, Brice Pitt's dictum of 'general psychiatry only more so' applies. The clinician treating an older adult with depression must take into account medical illness, multiple medical and psychotropic drugs, cognitive and neurologic factors, as well as the complex psychosocial history and milieu of the patient and their family.

B. Bipolar disorders and mania

Definition

Bipolar disorders are defined by the history or presence of a manic or hypomanic episode as defined by DSM-IV as outlined in Table 7.3.

Table 7.3 DSM-IV criteria for manic episode.

Manic episode

A. A distinct period of abnormally and persistently elevated, expansive, or irritable mood, lasting at least one week (or any duration if hospitalization is necessary).

B. During the period of mood disturbance, three (or more) of the following symptoms have persisted (four if the mood is only irritable) and have been present to a significant degree:

   (1) inflated self-esteem or grandiosity;

   (2) decreased need for sleep (e.g. feels rested after only three hours of sleep);

   (3) more talkative than usual or pressure to keep talking;

   (4) flight of ideas or subjective experience that thoughts are racing;

   (5) distractibility (i.e. attention too easily drawn to unimportant or irrelevant external stimuli);

   (6) increase in goal-directed activity (either socially, at work or school, or sexually) or psychomotor agitation;

   (7) excessive involvement in pleasurable activities that have a high potential for painful consequences (e.g. engaging in unrestrained buying sprees, sexual indiscretions, or foolish business investments).

C. The symptoms do not meet criteria for a mixed episode.

D. The mood disturbance is sufficiently severe to cause marked impairment in occupational functioning or in usual social activities or relationships with others, or to necessitate hospitalization to prevent harm to self or others, or there are psychotic features.

E. The symptoms are not due to the direct physiological effects of a substance (e.g. a drug of abuse, a medication, or other treatment) or a general medical condition (e.g. hyperthyroidism).

Hypomanic episode

The episode is not severe enough to cause marked impairment in social or occupational functioning, or to necessitate hospitalization, and there are no psychotic features.

Special considerations

Bipolar disorder in later life is still a relatively uncommon disorder and, from a public health perspective, carries less import than the more prevalent depressive spectrum of disorders. Despite its relative rarity, the study of bipolar disorder in later life does have heuristic value in order to understand why older patients become manic late in life compared to the more common early-onset bipolar patients, and in turn compared to age-matched depression patients. Unfortunately, the current state of knowledge is based primarily on retrospective cohort studies, case reports, small case series and only recently from epidemiological data using large health databases.

Classification

The high levels of medical and neurological co-morbidity in the elderly bipolar population have clouded the diagnostic picture. This has been complicated by the classification of DSM-IV which includes a category of 'mood disorder due to a general medical condition (293.83)'. This diagnosis implies that 'the disturbance is the direct physiologic consequences of a general medical condition'. Unfortunately, the high levels of co-morbidity prevalent in later life make the assumption of 'direct physiologic consequence' very difficult to ascertain. The assumption of an aetiological relationship is most precarious in these circumstances.

An earlier classification, known as 'secondary mania', implied that the systemic medical factors were responsible for this syndrome. Supporting evidence includes a close temporal relationship between medical/neurologic conditions and the manic syndrome. A negative family history is further support of this subtype. Others have suggested that mania in late life resembles the neurologically defined 'disinhibition syndrome'. Affective vulnerability, be it acquired or genetic, may have been expressed in earlier life as a temperamental vulnerability. However, cerebral–organic factors may unmask this vulnerability and produce what psychiatrists classify as a 'manic syndrome'.

Epidemiology

It is important to distinguish between the prevalence of bipolar disorder based on hospital admission rates compared to community-based surveys. For in-patient psychogeriatric units, a relatively high 'treated prevalence' of 8% has been reported. Furthermore, first admission rates for mania show a modest increase at the extremes of late life. Indeed, specialized psychogeriatric units report approximately 7–10 admissions per year. This relatively high prevalence of manic and bipolar disorders sits in stark contrast to community studies, such as the Epidemiologic Catchment Area (ECA) study, which showed a negligible prevalence of mania in the over 60s who were living in the community (<0.1%). This is dramatically lower than the relatively high prevalence of 1.4% found in young adults. This discrepancy in community prevalence begs the question 'where have all the young bipolars gone?'. A number of theories have been posited, including the relatively high mortality rate from natural causes, an increased rate of suicide and a suggestion that in the longer term, bipolarity 'burns out'. These questions remain unanswered and may only be addressed through carefully designed prospective studies of long duration.

Age of onset

Age of onset remains an important variable in distinguishing subtypes of bipolarity, which in turn may reflect a different pathogenesis and aetiology. For elderly bipolar patients, the median age of onset tends to be around age 50 and this is emerging as the most commonly used cut-off point for 'late-onset' disease.

One-year incidence rates in Finland revealed that almost 20% of first admissions for bipolar disorder occur after the age of 60. In stark contrast, community-based samples, such as the ECA study and the US National Co-morbidity Study

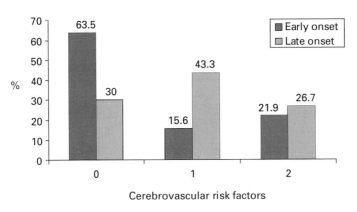

Geriatric bipolar disorder

Figure 7.1 The relationship between cerebrovascular disorders and the risk of mania. Adapted from Wylie, M.E. *et al.* (1999).

(see further reading section below) report a mean age of onset for bipolar disorder in the early 20s.

Using age 50 as the cut-off for a late-onset group of elderly bipolar patients, a significant increase in cerebrovascular risk factors was found by Wylie *et al.* (see 1999 article in the further reading section below) (see Figure 7.1). This is not dissimilar to findings in elderly depressed patients where vascular depression and other vascular risk factors have emerged as very significant contributing factors and co-morbid phenomena. Even with late-onset subjects who have a lesser family history of psychiatric disorders compared to early-onset cases, the prevalence of positive family history in first-degree relatives of elderly bipolar patients remains higher than the general population. Moreover, older bipolar patients have greater genetic loading than control groups with major depression only.

Neurological co-morbidity and pathophysiology

The high prevalence of co-morbid neurological disease in older bipolar patients has been a robust finding over many studies using different populations. The neurologic co-morbidity has led the neurologic literature to use the terms 'disinhibition syndrome' and 'secondary mania'. Moreover, pathological laughing and crying which may or may not be related to mood disorders, such as depression and mania, tend to differentiate by lesion location. Pathological laughing is associated with right-sided lesions, while left-sided lesions tend to produce pathologic crying.

The underlying pathophysiology for bipolarity may relate to the integrity of the frontal, limbic and basal ganglia circuitry, known functionally as the orbitofrontal circuit. This integrates sensory input with motivational states. Evidence primarily from the neuroimaging literature supports the hypothesis that right-sided orbitofrontal lesions mediate manic syndromes. Furthermore, a preponderance of basal temporal lesions was found in the first year following head injury (see the Jorge *et al.*, 1993 article in the further reading section below). Patients with frontotemporal dementia, distinct from AD, present with disinhibition phenomena that may mimic mania. This is an important differential diagnostic issue, but may be also relevant to understanding the underlying pathophysiology for more typical bipolar disorders. For example, in cases of dementia with disinhibition, there was a greater decrease in metabolic activity in the orbitofrontal circuit than in parietal areas. It may be that secondary mania results from disinhibition produced by lesions that disrupt connections within the orbitofrontal circuit. Frontal lobes modulate motivational and psychomotor behaviour while limbic connections modulate emotions. Furthermore, the biogenic amine nuclei located in the amygdala, brainstem and hypothalamus may in turn modulate instinctive behaviours that are connected to the syndrome of mania.

More support for lesion location comes from a review of focal unilateral cortical lesions (see the article by Braun *et al.*, 1999 in the further reading section). Right-sided lesions tend to produce mania and 'pseudomania', whereas left-hemisphere lesions tend to be associated with depression and 'pseudodepression'.

The extent of neurological co-morbidity has been approximated in retrospective studies of late-life bipolarity. Neurological co-morbidity was 36% in manic patients compared to only 8% in age- and sex-matched patients with depression. Within the manic sub-group, a first affective episode of mania late in life was more likely to be associated with a neurological lesion (71%) compared to those elderly patients who experienced multiple episodes by the time they had reached old age.

The most common neurological disorder described in the literature is cerebrovascular disease. Similar to the vascular depression hypothesis, a vascular subtype of mania has been proposed. This subtype is based on clinical and neuroimaging findings of cerebrovascular disease. Supporting clinical evidence includes a history of stroke, transient ischaemic attack (TIA) or focal signs, while positive neuroimaging includes the presence of hyperintensities or silent cerebral infarctions. Certainly, cognitive dysfunction is more common in this sub-group.

Neuroimaging

Sub-cortical hyperintensities predominate in studies of bipolar disorder, especially in later life. These sub-cortical hyperintensities have been assumed to reflect cerebrovascular disease. This includes hypertension, arteriosclerotic heart disease and diabetes mellitus. Late-onset mania has also been associated with a higher than expected prevalence of silent cerebral infarctions as found on neuroimaging. These patients tend to have a lower incidence of family history in first-degree relatives which supports the 'vascular mania' hypothesis.

Clinical course and outcome

Elderly bipolar patients experience the onset of a mood disorder at a mean of 50 years, the accepted cut-off for 'late onset'. Half the index patients who are first hospitalized for depression then demonstrate a strikingly long latency (mean 15 years) prior to the onset of their first manic episode and switch to a bipolar diagnosis. Of this sub-group, approximately one-quarter have a latency of at least 25 years until first mania. This 'conversion' to a bipolar diagnosis after many years of unipolar depression is strongly suggestive of the role that cerebral organic factors and co-morbid neurologic disorders play in late-life bipolar disorder.

Even though a diagnosis of bipolar disorder hinges on the presence of a single episode of mania, the vast majority of elderly bipolar patients experience a clinical course with both depressive and manic episodes. Only a small sub-group (12%) meet strict criteria for a course of unipolar mania. This sub-group has an age of onset that is significantly lower compared to the larger group of elderly manic patients. Indeed, the unipolar manic patients are among the very few elderly affective disorder patients whose illness tended to begin early in life, suggesting a unique pathogenesis.

Outcome of bipolar disorder in late life carries a significant morbidity and mortality. In one study, half of hospitalized elderly manic patients had died at a mean six-year follow-up compared to only 20% of elderly depressed patients. Furthermore, others have found manic patients to suffer from greater morbidity including cognitive dysfunction, cerebrovascular disease and to have a poor prognosis.

The determinants of bipolar disorder in later life

1. Notwithstanding a general pattern that suggests a lower genetic loading in later-onset disorders of all types, the bipolar sub-group in late life still carries a significant familial prevalence of mood disorder (50–85%) in first-degree relatives. However, the issue of familial affective vulnerability may be based not only on genetic factors, but on the psychological events of early life. Given the ubiquitous presence of losses in later life, it may very well be that the more important losses related to bipolarity in late life are those that occur early in an individual's development.

2. The conversion of a latent bipolar disorder after many years suggests the contribution of degenerative changes associated with normal ageing. However, the neuroimaging literature in retrospective studies points to heterogeneous brain lesions with a predominance of cerebrovascular disease associated with mania late in life. Other conditions that have been implicated include a variety of brain tumours, chronic alcoholism and a wide range of metabolic conditions.

3. Finally, the vulnerability to mood disorder and the presence of brain changes may not be sufficient to produce a relatively uncommon syndrome such as mania in later life. The localization of those lesions to the right hemisphere

and specifically to the orbitofrontal circuit may be the critical factor in the manifestation of this relatively uncommon condition. Thus, localization of brain pathology to the right-sided orbitofrontal circuit, in combination with a vulnerability to mood disorder, may constitute the pathogenetic combination necessary for the development of mania in late life.

Treatment

There have been no randomized controlled trials of pharmacological treatment in an older bipolar patient population. Consequently, clinicians need to rely on guidelines that are designed for mixed-age populations and extrapolate from the evidence available on pharmacokinetic and pharmacodynamic changes in older adults. Atypical neuroleptics are generally favoured for the acute severe manic episode, although recent efficacy studies show value for atypicals in the continuation phase. Mood stabilizers may be introduced in the acute phase and are continued for longer periods of prophylaxis.

Lithium carbonate remains the mainstay of pharmacological treatment for bipolar disorder in all ages and this should be the same in an older population. However, there are special considerations regarding the use of lithium in old age, primarily related to the fact that lithium is eliminated exclusively by the kidneys. Hence, age-associated decreases in creatinine clearance and lithium clearance affect serum lithium levels. Furthermore, pharmacodynamic factors cause an increased vulnerability to adverse reactions in an older population. Specifically, the use of drugs such as diuretics, angiotensin converting enzyme (ACE inhibitors) and non-steroidal anti-inflammatory drugs (NSAIDs) have been implicated in cases of lithium toxicity and have been shown to increase serum levels of lithium. This is a significant concern because these drugs are so commonly prescribed to older adults. Notwithstanding the appropriate cautions associated with the use of lithium carbonate in older adults, lithium has remained a standard treatment for a large cohort of bipolar patients. Sudden discontinuation of lithium carbonate at any age, and especially in old age, is very likely to result in a significant relapse of the bipolar condition.

Recent pharmacoepidemiological data show a dramatic decrease in prescription patterns for lithium compared to sodium valproate/divalproex in older adults with new-onset bipolar disorder. It would appear that marketing factors combined with concerns about the potential toxicity of lithium carbonate have favoured this shift in clinical practice. Unfortunately, there is little evidence to support this trend in terms of effectiveness or safety data. For example, a population-based cohort study found no significant difference between the incidence of delirium in older adults treated for the first time with lithium compared to sodium valproate/divalproex. However, as has been known previously, new treatment with lithium carbonate in older adults is indeed associated with a significant increase in the development of hypothyroidism requiring thyroxine replacement therapy (approximately 6% per annum).

Despite the potential difficulties and adverse events associated with lithium carbonate in older adults, the dramatic change in prescription patterns should be reconsidered in light of its longstanding use as a mainstay treatment for bipolar disorder. In the meantime, careful monitoring of older patients on lithium is essential. Unfortunately, guidelines for serum levels are problematic in that we have little scientific basis by which to monitor serum levels, although it is clear that the usual therapeutic range for younger adult populations (0.5–1.2 mmol/l) is inappropriate for an older population. Clinical consensus suggests that the maintenance serum lithium level should be closer to 0.5 mmol/l with a maximum in the 0.8 mmol/l range, above which serious side effects become very likely.

Other mood stabilizing agents, such as carbamazepine, lamotrigine and oxcarbazepine, have shown promising results in mixed-age bipolar patients but have not yet been studied in a systematic manner in older adults. Similarly, a number of atypical antipsychotic agents such as olanzapine, risperidone, arapiprazole and quetiapine have shown efficacy in a mixed-age bipolar population, especially for the treatment of mania and in continuation therapy. However, there are very few data on an older population.

As highlighted in Chapter 2, the involvement of carers and family members in the management of bipolar disorder in older adults is especially important. Like all major psychiatric disorders, the family is profoundly affected by bipolarity and deserves attention in the management of these disorders. Caregivers can guide treatment, and in turn psychoeducation for family members may improve adherence.

Summary

Bipolar disorder in older adults, as defined by an episode of mania or hypomania, represents a prototypic neuropsychiatric syndrome which in turn reflects its neurologic basis. None the less, affective vulnerability (usually genetic, sometimes psychological) is associated with the late manifestation of mania, often precipitated by heterogeneous neurologic disorders. Cerebrovascular pathology is particularly common as evidenced clinically as well as on neuroimaging by lacunar infarcts, cortical and sub-cortical hyperintensities. The localization of these brain lesions to the right side of the brain affecting the orbitofrontal circuit appears to be specific to late-onset mania. Treatment of bipolarity in old age must take into account the significant co-morbidity and special considerations, including decreased renal function associated with long-term lithium therapy, which has been the mainstay of bipolar treatment of the last generation. Newer pharmacological agents, including the atypical neuroleptics and the anticonvulsant class of drugs, offer a variety of alternatives that require more formal evaluation in an older population. Involvement of family remains an essential component of ongoing management.

FURTHER READING

Articles

Alexopoulos, G. S. (2005). Depression in the elderly. *Lancet,* **365**, 1961–1970.
Clear overview from one of the most highly respected researchers in the field.

Almeida, O. (2008). Vascular depression: myth or reality? *International Psychogeriatrics,* **20**, 645–652.
An impassioned refutation of the vascular depression hypothesis.

Baldwin, R. *et al.* (2005). Neurological findings in late-onset depressive disorder: comparison of individuals with and without depression. *British Journal of Psychiatry,* **186**, 308–313.
Important paper suggesting a difference in the prevalence of neurologic disorders between depressed and non-depressed elderly people.

Baldwin, R. C. and O'Brien, J. (2002). Vascular basis of late-onset depressive disorder. *British Journal of Psychiatry,* **180**, 157–160.
Evidence-based argument in favour of the vascular depression hypothesis.

Braun, C. M. J. *et al.* (1999). Mania, pseudomania, depression, and pseudodepression resulting from focal unilateral cortical lesions. *Neuropsychiatry, Neuropsychology and Behavioral Neurology,* **12**, 35–51.
Evidence to suggest that brain injury is an important predeterminant of some late-life affective syndromes.

Jorge, R. E. *et al.* (1993). Secondary mania following traumatic brain injury. *American Journal of Psychiatry,* **150**, 916–921.
Kessler R. C. *et al.* (1997). The epidemiology of DSM-IIIR bipolar I disorder in a general population survey. *Psychological Medicine,* **27**, 1079–1089.
Data from the ECA study.

Krauthammer, C. and Klerman, G. L. (1978). Secondary mania: manic syndromes associated with antecedent physical illness or drugs. *Archives of General Psychiatry,* **35**, 1333–1339.
Evidence for the association of manic syndromes with prior illness or drug use.

Mottram, P., Wilson, K. and Strobl, J. (2006). Antidepressants for depressed elderly (Review). In: The Cochrane Library, Issue 1. *The Cochrane Collaboration* (pp. 1–52). Chichester: John Wiley and Sons, Ltd. http://www.thecochranelibrary.com.
Mulsant, B. H. *et al.* (2003). Achieving long-term optimal outcomes in geriatric depression and anxiety. *CNS Spectrum,* **8**, 27–34.
Addresses the important issue of prophylaxis.

Shulman, K. I. *et al.* (1992). Mania compared with unipolar depression in old age. *American Journal of Psychiatry,* **142**, 341–345.
Useful comparative paper.

Shulman K. I. *et al.* (2003). Changing prescription patterns for lithium and divalproex in old age: shifting practice without evidence. *BMJ,* **326**, 960–961.
Evidence-based argument in favour of the continued use of lithium for prophylaxis in bipolar disorders.

Wylie, M. E. *et al.* (1999). Age at onset in geriatric bipolar disorder. *American Journal of Geriatric Psychiatry, 7,* 77–83.
As noted above, this paper examines the issue of age of onset.

Book chapters

Baldwin, R. (2008). Depressive disorders. In R. Jacoby, C. Oppenheimer, T. Dening and A. Thomas, (Eds.) *The Oxford Textbook of Old Age Psychiatry* (pp. 529–556). Oxford: Oxford University Press.
A masterly summary of the existing literature.

Shulman, K. I. and Herrmann, N. (2008). Manic syndromes in old age. In R. Jacoby, C. Oppenheimer, T. Dening and A. Thomas, (Eds.) *The Oxford Textbook of Old Age Psychiatry* (pp. 563–572). Oxford: Oxford University Press.
This chapter offers a more detailed overview of mania and related issues than can be provided in a short text.

Weissman, M. M. *et al.* (1991). Affective disorders. In L. N. Robins and D. A. Regier, (Eds.) *Psychiatric Disorders in America: the Epidemiologic Catchment Area Study* (pp. 53–90). New York, NY: Free Press.
A report from a very influential epidemiological study.

8

Schizophrenia and related disorders in late life

Brief historical notes

Most mental health professionals have some familiarity with the diagnosis of schizophrenia and psychoses occurring in young adults. For people with psychosis in late life, the term 'late paraphrenia' had some currency from the 1950s until around 10 years ago.

Kraepelin, in his introduction to his classic text *Dementia Praecox and Paraphrenia* (English translation 1919) distinguished between dementia praecox and paraphrenia which he described thus: 'those forms have been singled out and placed together subsequently which are distinguished in their whole course by very definite manifestations of peculiar disturbances of intellect while lacking enfeeblement of volition and especially of feeling, or at least such symptoms are only feebly indicated. It seems to be that the term "paraphrenia", which is now no longer in common use, is in the meantime suitable as the name of morbid forms thus delimited which are here by way of experiment brought together'.

In the UK, the term 'late paraphrenia' was introduced in the 1950s by Roth to describe some schizophrenia-like conditions first appearing in those over the age of 60. This term was current up to the International Classification of Diseases, Version 9 (ICD-9) (1980), but was not included in Version 10 (ICD-10) (1993).

Since the 1960s, there has been much discussion and debate regarding the nature and classification of late-onset psychosis, the central issues being as follows:

(a) Is this the same as schizophrenia in the young adult but occurring later in the elderly?

(b) Is this biologically similar or different to schizophrenia in the younger adult?

(c) Is late-onset psychosis a result of the interaction between schizophrenia and the multiple vulnerability factors associated with old age?

(d) Is late paraphrenia the end product of an ongoing psychosis?

To address these issues and resolve the controversy, an international consensus meeting was held at Leeds Castle, Kent, UK in July 1998. It resulted in the following consensus statement agreed by the expert participants:

The term paraphrenia is best dropped. Non-organic, non-affective psychoses that have a first onset in late life can be divided epidemiologically into three categories:

(a) Late-onset schizophrenia (LOS) (illness onset after 40 years of age but otherwise indistinguishable from schizophrenia starting at an earlier age) and,

(b) Very-late-onset schizophrenia-like psychosis (VLOSP) (onset after 60 years). This latter group is generally associated with a somewhat different symptom profile and does not seem to have genetic risk factors for schizophrenia.

Early-onset schizophrenia: the evolution of this disorder with advancing age

Kraepelin conceptualized inevitable and inexorable deterioration in personality and psychosocial functioning as being a core part of dementia praecox (later renamed as schizophrenia by Bleuler). However, long-term studies have identified that although schizophrenia can be chronic, disabling and with outcome worse than other mental disorders, improvement and/or recovery can occur in half to two-thirds of cases. The movement towards de-institutionalization, and the ageing of the 'baby boomer' cohort, will result in more 'graduates' (people with life-long schizophrenia who have grown old) living in the community requiring treatment, support and management from specialist old-age psychiatry services.

The ongoing psychotic symptoms of chronic schizophrenia in old age are usually a continuation of what has appeared in the patient's earlier younger years – delusions, hallucinations (usually auditory), and thought disorder. These may be attenuated in intensity and frequency by time. The ageing process, in entering developmental maturity, may exert an ameliorating affect on the symptoms.

However, ongoing negative symptoms of avolition, blunted affect, deterioration of personality and psychosocial function, such as described by Kraepelin, may, when present, become more severe. The confounding effects of depression, psychosocial isolation resulting from many years of negative symptomatology combined with demoralization, lack of social support, long periods of hospitalization, and continuous use of antipsychotic medication negatively impact on their quality of life and thus make negative symptoms appear to be more severe and disabling.

The emergence of cognitive impairment in old age will further compound these problems, thus creating a 'double jeopardy'. Although some old people with schizophrenia may be entering a dementing process, it is to be noted that not all cognitive impairment in these patients represents dementia and may be due to incident delirium, the cognitive symptoms of schizophrenia itself, or other causes such as medication use or depression.

Schizophrenia with onset in late life

As many studies in late-life schizophrenia were done prior to the Leeds Castle consensus meeting, and only a few have been published in the short span of time since 1998, our knowledge of the condition which that meeting defined as VLOSP is only slowly emerging.

Table 8.1 Clinical presentation of schizophrenia in late life. (Reproduced with permission from Hassett, A., Ames, D., and Chiu E. (2005). *Psychosis in the Elderly*. London: Taylor and Francis).

Early onset	Late onset
Delusions	Delusions
• systematized	• systematized
• non-systematized	• 'partition'
	• phantom boarders
Hallucinations	Hallucinations
• usually auditory	• multi-modal
Thought disorder	Thought disorder
• common	• uncommon
Negative symptoms	Negative symptoms
• common	• uncommon

Clinical features

Phenomenologically, delusions and hallucinations can emerge for the first time at any age; other features of schizophrenia, such as thought disorder, affective blunting, and avolition appear to become less frequent with increasing age. 'Partition' delusions (relating to the phantom presence of hallucinatory voices or noises emanating from the floors, ceilings or walls of one's abode) with persecutory themes are more prominent in old age. Table 8.1 summarizes the contrasting presentations.

Epidemiology

While there are multiple methodological issues in studies reporting epidemiological data in late-onset schizophrenia, nevertheless a general picture can be obtained.

The Ageing and Liverpool Health Aspects Study with a sample of 5222 community subjects reported a prevalence of 0.12%. The Epidemiological Catchment Area (ECA) study in the USA reported a one-year prevalence rate of 0.6% in subjects between 45 and 64 years and 0.2% for those over 65 years.

There is a strong predominance of females in late-onset schizophrenia ranging from a high 22.5:1 female:male ratio to a low 1.6:1, suggesting a particular vulnerability in women for first onset of a psychotic illness in late life.

Risk factors, apart from the obvious genetic factors, include the contribution of sensory impairment, social isolation and premorbid personality with prominent paranoid/schizoid traits.

Neuroimaging in late-onset schizophrenia (LOS)

To try to understand the pathological processes in the development of LOS and VLOSP, neuroimaging is potentially a most useful tool in studies of this condition.

However, at this stage of neuroimaging technology and research, the findings in LOS are similar to that of early-onset schizophrenia (EOS), which include increased Ventricular Brain Ratio (VBR), and reduction in Regional Blood Flow (RBF) in the temporal area. The role of white matter hyperintensities (WMHs) is unclear. The new technologies of fMRI, magnetic resonance spectroscopy (MRS) and MEG (magnetoencephalography) may in the future help elucidate possible aetiologies in late-onset schizophrenia.

Cognitive change in late-onset schizophrenia

Cognitive impairment is part of the clinical characteristics of schizophrenia, both in EOS and LOS, and is generally similar. The cognitive impairment is static and occasionally reversible with treatment. This contrasts with that of neurodegenerative disorders such as dementia.

Neuropsychological studies have demonstrated that LOS is not associated with senile plaques or obvious amyloid pathology, suggesting that the neuropathological processes of LOS and AD are not the same.

There is no evidence of a disproportionately higher rate of cognitive decline or dementia amongst LOS subjects.

Management of late-onset schizophrenia and 'graduates' with long standing early-onset schizophrenia

Physical management

As medical co-morbidity is the rule rather than the exception in late life, the identification and energetic treatment of such conditions is a priority. The management of general physical health will benefit all patients with schizophrenia. The collaboration of a family physician and/or specialist geriatricians/physicians will enhance this aspect of management.

'Graduates' who have been disabled by schizophrenia for many years may have neglected their physical health and may not have had consistent health maintenance. Therefore close attention should be given to this aspect in assessment and any outstanding issues should be actively pursued.

For those who develop schizophrenia in late life, and who have had good health maintenance up to date, this should be encouraged to be continued.

Pharmacological management

For 'graduates' who are continuing their pharmacological management, consistent and constant monitoring of compliance, adverse effects and the interaction with other drugs should be a high priority. Any change of medication will need to take into consideration the alteration in physiological status of an elderly person and the effects on development of adverse events. At least one study has shown that patients on classical antipsychotics whose symptoms are not well controlled or who experience significant side effects from these medications may benefit when their treatment is switched to olanzapine or risperidone.

To start treatment for LOS and particularly VLOSP, atypical antipsychotics (olanzapine, risperidone, quetiapine, aripiprazole, etc.) are the drugs of choice. The efficacy of these medications has been adequately demonstrated in trials including younger patients, but there is a paucity of data to guide the prescriber whose patients are elderly. They do reduce core schizophrenic symptoms, have low extra-pyramidal side effects, and are much better tolerated than conventional (typical) antipsychotics. The choice between available atypical antipsychotics is not at all clear and there is little evidence to support the use of one over the other in relation to efficacy or the emergence of such adverse effects as motor disorders, although each has marginal and different adverse events in other domains. Doses prescribed should be as low as possible (e.g. 1–4 mg risperidone daily, 2.5–15 mg olanzapine daily), while achieving a therapeutic effect. In practice the optimum dose to be used will need to be determined for each patient, with factors such as symptom control and the presence of dose-dependent adverse effects being pre-eminent. Some patients will do poorly on one drug and better on another. Not every patient will respond to treatment; studies of classical antipsychotics suggest that one-quarter to one-third of patients with LOS and VLOSP receive no net benefit from antipsychotic therapy, and only one-quarter achieve complete remission. Nevertheless, even a modest amelioration of symptoms may allow a supervised return to independent living in the community.

Psychosocial management

The psychosocial needs of this group of patients who are increasingly living independently in the community highlight the necessity to develop multidisciplinary comprehensive management strategies to improve their quality of life in conjunction with effective symptom reduction through energetic pharmacological treatment.

As they have multiple, complex needs, resulting from a combination of physical psychological and psychotic symptoms in late life, the strategies of case management combined with individual service plans in consultation with the patient and any significant family members should underpin their care. This will provide holistic and comprehensive support taking care of all the psychosocial and physical aspects of their lives.

Residential care

As they age and functional capacity declines, consideration for residential care would require careful consultation to achieve the best quality of life at this latter stage of their lives.

Table 8.2 Psychotic symptoms across life stages. (Reproduced with permission from Hassett, A., Ames, D., and Chiu, E. (2005). *Psychosis in the Elderly*. London: Taylor and Francis).

	Young	Middle age	Old age
Schizophrenia	+	+	+
Affective disorders	+	+	++
Alcohol misuse	+	++	+
Illicit substance use	++	+	
Delusional disorder		+	+
Specific organic		+	++
Delirium			++
Dementia			++

As most residential care services for the older person are planned for frail elderly and those with dementia as the major consumer groups, elderly patients with schizophrenia may not be appropriately located in such facilities. Special consideration will need to be made for this group of patients requiring residential care. The development of specialist psychogeriatric nursing homes such as those that exist in Victoria, Australia, to cater for this group of patients may be a model to be considered.

Other conditions which may exhibit psychotic symptoms (also see Chapters 5–7 and 10)

Psychotic symptoms occurring for the first time in late life frequently pose a diagnostic and management dilemma for the clinician. Table 8.2 illustrates a comparison of psychotic symptoms across life stages.

Psychotic symptoms occur frequently in elderly people with delirium. This is usually under-recognized and not given adequate weight in DSM-IV, which did not include delusions as one of the features of delirium.

Elderly people with depressive illnesses can also present with psychotic symptoms, which may be mood-congruent, with the content of delusions and hallucinations being consistent with the depressive themes of guilt, personal deprecation, nihilism or deserved punishment for exaggerated past sins. Mania, whether it is part of an ongoing primary bipolar disorder or secondary to pathology related to central nervous system disorders, can include psychotic features of grandiose delusions, inappropriate sexual expression and paranoid response if prevented from acting out behaviours resulting from these psychotic symptoms.

Psychotic features in dementia are well-recognized and have been extensively researched (see Chapter 5). In elderly persons presenting with psychotic symptoms for the first time, dementia should always be kept in mind and explored vigorously.

The presence of psychotic symptoms in specific neurological disorders such as basal ganglia disorders (especially Parkinson's disease) and cerebrovascular disease should be noted. Adverse psychotic reactions to drugs used to treat Parkinson's disease occur quite frequently.

Iatrogenic substance-induced causes of psychotic symptoms

One of the very common causes of psychotic symptoms in the elderly is the adverse effect of both prescribed and over-the-counter preparations. Anticholinergic drugs, dopamine agonists, opiates, corticosteroids, tricyclic antidepressants, low-potency conventional antipsychotics, non-steroidal inflammatory drugs, and digoxin are well known high-risk drugs for the causation of delirium and psychotic features in the elderly. Benzodiazepines, beta-blocking drugs and calcium channel blocking agents have lower, but nevertheless significant, risks attached to their use.

Medication monitoring and constant review by clinicians is an essential best practice in the management of all elderly patients.

Conclusion

While the concept and classification of schizophrenia is still under continuing review, nevertheless, the distress of psychotic symptoms to the elderly and their families should cause all clinicians to take the greatest care in the identification and management of these symptoms, whether they be due to schizophrenic spectrum disorders or to other possible causes in the elderly.

FURTHER READING

Articles

Howard, R. *et al.* (2000). Late onset schizophrenia – very late onset schizophrenia-like psychosis: an international consensus. *American Journal of Psychiatry,* **157**, 172–178.
The current international consensus on classifying this complex group of disorders.

Jeste, D. V. *et al.* (1999). Conventional versus newer antipsychotics in the elderly. *American Journal of Geriatric Psychiatry,* 7, 70–76.
A balanced view of the pharmacological treatment options.

Ritchie, C. *et al.* (2003). The impact upon extra-pyramidal side effects, clinical symptoms and quality of life of a switch from conventional to atypical antipsychotics (Risperidone or Olanzapine) in elderly patients with schizophrenia. *International Journal of Geriatric Psychiatry,* **18**, 432–440.

Ritchie, C. *et al.* (2006). A comparison of the efficacy and safety of olanzapine and risperidone in the treatment of elderly patients with schizophrenia: an open study of six months duration. *International Journal of Geriatric Psychiatry*, **21**, 171–179.

These two papers offer supportive evidence for the safety and efficacy of switching the treatment of elderly patients with schizophrenia from conventional antipsychotics to olanzapine or risperidone.

Book

Hassett, A., Ames, D., and Chiu, E. (2005). *Psychosis in the Elderly*. London: Taylor and Francis.

A detailed and comprehensive overview of all forms of psychosis affecting the elderly.

Book chapter

Howard, R. (2008). Late onset schizophrenia and very late onset schizophrenia-like psychosis. In R. Jacoby, C. Oppenheimer, T. Dening and A. Thomas, (Eds.) *Oxford Textbook of Old Age Psychiatry* (pp. 519–572). Oxford: Oxford University Press.

A superb, historically informed overview of schizophrenia and related disorders in late life by the leading expert in the field.

9

Neurotic and personality disorders

A. NEUROTIC DISORDERS

Introduction

Neurotic disorders are characterized by the psychological and somatic symptoms of anxiety and depression, complicated by various maladaptive attempts to manage and control these symptoms, such as phobic avoidance and somatization. These conditions are the commonest mental disorders at all ages, and they incur substantial direct and indirect costs to health and social services. Despite the fact that neurotic disorders are relatively prevalent in the elderly population, they tend not to present to services, or else are missed or misdiagnosed if they do. This is a pity, because in many cases they are significantly distressing and disabling, and they are potentially treatable.

The concept of neurosis

The unitary and dimensional concept of neurosis that developed over the eighteenth and nineteenth centuries has given way in the modern era to a wide range of discretely defined categorical disorders, currently enshrined in the ICD-10 and DSM-IV classifications (Table 9.1). This categorical approach to illness is congenial to the modern case-oriented way of medical thinking, involving as it does decision-making, discriminating, service planning, and the organizing of reimbursement and research. However, it does not follow therefore that all forms of illness conform to this model, and there is good evidence that neurotic disorders are related to each other in important and fundamental ways. For example, there is extensive co-morbidity between this group of disorders and between them and depression, and follow-up studies demonstrate that there is also considerable movement of individuals between these diagnostic categories with the passage of time. Perhaps most importantly, diagnosis does not appear to be particularly helpful in predicting response to specific forms of treatment. What the two-dimensional categories of ICD-10 and DSM-IV fail to capture is the reality of common mental disorders as processes, the complex and variable outcome of interactions between individual vulnerability, circumstances, and inappropriate and self-defeating responses to distress. This is particularly important for understanding elderly patients, who often come with a lifetime's experience of their condition and its consequences.

Table 9.1 Current classifications of neurotic disorders.

ICD-10	DSM-IV
MOOD DISORDERS	MOOD DISORDERS
F34: *Persistent mood disorders*	DEPRESSIVE DISORDERS
Dysthymia	300.4: Dysthymic disorder
NEUROTIC, STRESS-RELATED AND SOMATOFORM DISORDERS	
F40: *Phobic anxiety disorders*	ANXIETY DISORDERS
.0: Agoraphobia	300.01: Panic disorder without agoraphobia
.1: Social phobia	300.21: Panic disorder with agoraphobia
.2: Specific phobia	300.22: Agoraphobia without history of panic disorder
F41: Other anxiety disorders	300.23: Social phobia
	300.29: Specific phobia
.0: Panic disorder	300.3: Obsessive–compulsive disorder
.1: Generalized anxiety disorder	309.81: Post-traumatic stress disorder
.2: Mixed anxiety and depressive disorder	300.02: Generalized anxiety disorder
	293.89: Anxiety disorder due to a general medical condition
F42: *Obsessive–compulsive disorder*	292.89: Substance-induced anxiety disorder
F43: *Reaction to severe stress, and adjust-ment disorders*	
.0: Acute stress reaction	
.1: Post-traumatic stress disorder	
.2: Adjustment disorders	
F44: *Dissociative disorders*	DISSOCIATIVE DISORDERS
.0: Dissociative amnesia	300.12: Dissociative amnesia
.1: Dissociative fugue	300.13: Dissociative fugue
.2: Dissociative stupor	300.14: Dissociative identity disorder
.3: Trance and possession states	300.6: Depersonalization disorder
.4: Dissociative motor disorders	
.5: Dissociative convulsions	
.6: Dissociative anaesthesia and sensory loss	
F45: *Somatoform disorders*	SOMATOFORM DISORDERS
.0: Somatization disorder	300.81: Somatization disorder
.1: Undifferentiated somatoform disorder	300.11: Conversion disorder
.2: Hypochondriacal disorder	300.7: Hypochondriasis
.3: Somatoform autonomic dysfunction	300.7: Body dysmorphic disorder
.4: Persistent somatoform pain disorder	307.80: Pain disorder associated with psychological factors
F46: *Other neurotic disorders*	307.89: Pain disorder associated with both psychological factors and a general medical condition
.0: Neurasthenia	
.1: Depersonalization–derealization	300.81: Undifferentiated somatoform syndrome disorder

The aetiology of neurotic disorders

According to Goldberg and Huxley (see the further reading section below for details of their influential 1992 text), all of the neurotic disorders are grounded in the core experiences of anxiety and depression, which in turn reflect the activity of specific neuronal systems in response to reward and punishment. A number of factors determine whether and when an individual develops an episode of illness, and the subsequent course of that episode.

Vulnerability factors

These determine an individual's general liability to develop psychological symptoms in response to adverse experiences. Genetic factors appear to have a diagnostically non-specific effect in increasing the risk of neurotic disorder, perhaps by determining emotional reactivity; the personality trait of 'neuroticism' is under a significant degree of genetic control. It has also been shown that across the lifespan, environmental and psychosocial factors such as early parental loss, limited education, chronic social adversity, poor social networks, low levels of social support and physical disability all increase vulnerability to neurotic disorders. Some factors, such as the impact of physical illness and disability, probably have a greater impact as vulnerability factors in older age groups. Environmental factors experienced during childhood may determine future vulnerability through their effect on personality development, in particular the favoured cognitive defence styles in the face of threat and loss. Factors experienced in adulthood, such as long standing social adversity, may act by increasing low self-esteem, or by increasing individuals' vulnerability to other factors, such as physical ill-health and other adverse life events.

Destabilization factors

These are the experiences that provoke the onset of psychological symptoms in sufficiently vulnerable individuals. The impact of adverse life events has been researched extensively at all ages, and it has been shown that experiences involving loss and threat are important in relation to the onset of depression and anxiety, respectively. It is the meaning of the event to the individual, not its objective severity, that matters most in terms of its liability to provoke illness. Some kinds of life event, such as retirement, bereavement, and institutionalization, occur more frequently in old age, and might therefore be important causes of anxiety and depression in this age group, but the evidence is by no means clear on this point. The 'timeliness' of such events in old age may reduce their impact, as may the degree of planning, preparation and choice involved.

Some extreme and catastrophic experiences, such as major accidents, war or natural disaster, have the potential to provoke significant psychological distress in all but the most robust individuals. In ICD-10 and DSM-IV, the close relationship between the trauma and the psychological response to it has led to these stress reactions being classified as separate diagnoses, notably post-traumatic stress disorder; they are discussed further below.

Restitution factors

These determine the duration of the psychological symptoms, and the nature of the recovery from them. Sometimes, the restitution from an episode of illness is uncomplicated, with individuals making a full recovery. Several factors contribute to successful restitution, including the nature of the episode (mild rather than severe), resolution of the provoking life event, crisis support, 'fresh start' events, and the lack of other complicating vulnerability factors, such as chronic social adversity and poor social networks. Mental health services can also contribute to the successful resolution of illness in many cases, as many of the randomized controlled trials of psychotropic drugs and psychological interventions against placebo have shown.

In some cases, the restitution from an episode of illness can be complicated by the development of damaging and disabling distress-management strategies, such as phobic avoidance, self-medication with alcohol and other drugs, re-labelling as physical illness, etc. If these persist, they can lead to the enduring clusters of symptoms and behaviour that we recognize as specific neurotic disorders (agoraphobia, somatization disorder, etc.).

Epidemiology

Comparisons between epidemiological studies are difficult, because the different rules employed with regard to symptom definition, severity and diagnostic hierarchies result in very different rates of these disorders. Some generally applicable findings from community population surveys include a fall in prevalence and incidence rates with increasing age across the adult lifespan, and a female preponderance for most disorders at all ages. Most elderly people with neurotic disorders developed them before their fifties, but elderly cases of phobic disorder, panic and obsessive–compulsive disorder (OCD) tend to be of later onset. Epidemiological studies have also identified a range of risk factors associated with neurotic disorders in elderly populations, such as female gender, ethnic group, physical illness and disability, and various markers of social adversity, such as dependency on state benefits.

Clinical features

The psychological and somatic symptoms and disturbances of behaviour associated with these disorders are broadly similar at all ages, but in elderly patients there may be differences in how they are expressed, or perceived by others. In this age group, the clinical challenge is to be appropriately alert to the possibility of neurotic disorder, without misattributing potentially significant and serious symptoms of underlying physical illness.

Psychological symptoms

As mentioned above, this group of disorders is characterised by an admixture of depressive and anxiety symptoms. Depressive symptomatology in late life is discussed in detail elsewhere (see Chapter 7). When other factors are taken into account, older people appear to worry less than younger people, but if they do it is more likely to be associated with mental disorder; significant worry in old age should therefore not be dismissed, but should prompt further assessment of the mental state. Similarly, clinically important fears expressed by elderly people are sometimes regarded as reasonable on the grounds of age alone; in fact, it is issues such as frailty and the availability of social support that are more important in determining these individuals' perceptions of vulnerability and risk.

The clinical features and phenomenology of OCD are also similar to those seen in younger patients. It is rare for OCD to have its onset in later life, although cases have been reported. More commonly, diagnoses of OCD made for the first time in old age are chronic disorders that have never been adequately assessed or treated (see below).

Somatic symptoms

The somatic symptoms of anxiety are also similar at all ages, and include autonomic symptoms, muscular tension pains and headaches, motor restlessness, dyspnoea, *globus hystericus* and the physical effects of hyperventilation. In elderly patients, however, there is much greater opportunity for misdiagnosis and unnecessary investigations; panic attacks are particularly prone to being referred on to cardiologists, neurologists and gastroenterologists. This probably contributes significantly to the burden of health care costs associated with these disorders in old age. There is also the difficulty of identifying and managing somatic anxiety symptoms in elderly patients with significant co-existing physical illness, such as individuals with chronic respiratory disease trapped in a vicious circle of anxiety and breathlessness. It is quite understandable why doctors should wish to investigate and refer elderly patients with unexplained physical symptoms; in view of the strong association between neurotic disorders and physical ill-health in old age, there is always the concern that there might be an important hidden physical cause. Some suggestions to guide clinical decision-making in this tricky area are given in the section on differential diagnosis below.

Somatization, or the expression of psychosocial distress in the form of physical symptoms, is a common phenomenon at all ages and in all cultures, and is the commonest means by which patients with a mental disorder present to primary health care. Despite the popular stereotype of the elderly patient preoccupied with their bowels or other bodily symptoms, it does not appear that somatization is in fact more prevalent in old age than in younger adulthood. In elderly psychiatric populations, it is particularly associated with anxiety and depression, and also with physical illness. It is usually managed by reassurance, and treatment of the underlying physical and psychological disorders. Most patients will understand and accept their misattribution of symptoms when this is explained, but a few do not; among these are individuals who meet criteria for a somatoform or somatisation disorder (see below).

Hysterical symptoms are an important exception to the general observation that the clinical significance of neurotic symptoms is similar in both younger and more elderly patients. As a rule, hysterical illness does not begin in old age. Apparently hysterical conversion reactions and dysmnesias are occasionally seen in elderly patients in response to stress, but such symptoms are usually due either to underlying undiagnosed physical illness, or to the release of dissociative tendencies in vulnerable personalities by organic cerebral pathology or functional psychiatric disorder.

Patients with clinically significant anxiety commonly present with complaints of delayed or interrupted sleep due to worry and nightmares. This may be more of a problem for elderly patients, whose sleep architecture is also subject to the normal age-related changes making sleep lighter and more prone to interruption. Individuals with sleep disturbance associated with a neurotic disorder are also prone to have difficulties with chronic hypnotic drug and alcohol use.

Behavioural disturbance

Most of the behavioural problems associated with anxiety and depression represent maladaptive attempts to control these unpleasant experiences (see restitution factors, above): phobic avoidance, substance abuse, cigarette smoking, deliberate self-harm, eating disorders, and the abnormal illness behaviour associated with somatization. In elderly patients with chronic neurotic disorders, these behavioural problems are likely to be of long standing and associated with significant adverse physical and psychological consequences. In some individuals with a past history of eating disorder or deliberate self-harm in early adulthood, the re-emergence of these problems in late life may indicate difficulty in adjusting to their old age.

Differential diagnosis

Depression

As we have seen, the origins of neurotic disorders and depression are closely related, and admixtures of depressive and anxiety symptoms are among the most frequent presentations, particularly in primary care settings. Therefore, the proper diagnostic question is not: 'is it depression or anxiety?', but: 'how much of each?'. Indeed, in elderly patients, the occurrence of generalized anxiety in the absence of significant depression is the exception rather than the rule. This has important implications for management, as the primary target for intervention may be the depression rather than the anxiety (see below).

Dementia

With the growth of memory clinics and the availability of antidementia drugs, increasing numbers of patients of all ages are being referred to specialist old-age psychiatry services with complaints of impairment in their cognitive function. A key diagnostic challenge in this group is to distinguish between organic and functional causes of this impairment. 'Pseudodementia' associated with a severe depressive illness is now well-recognized, but subjective cognitive inefficiency can also be caused by much milder levels of both depression and anxiety, and may well be the presenting complaint in some cases. This differential diagnosis is complicated by the fact that a dementia can sometimes be heralded by episodes of anxiety and depression. In some cases, detailed neuropsychological assessment can help by finding a pattern of impairment indicative of either a functional or an organic disorder, but it is not uncommon for both this and other investigations to be uninformative. In these patients, the best course of action is to treat the functional symptoms, establish optimum baseline cognitive functioning, and reassess this in a year.

A diagnosis of dementia is a major life event, and it is quite common for individuals to develop significant secondary symptoms of anxiety and depression, particularly in the early stages when insight is preserved. There is loss of confidence, worry about the future and about the family, increased irritability, and social withdrawal due to fear of humiliating lapses in public. Anxiety and depression may also be more directly due to the underlying cause of the dementia, such as cerebrovascular disease (q.v.).

Delirium

Delirium is usually a quiet disorder in elderly patients, but sometimes they present with a hyperactive profile including increased arousal, irritability, and fear and aggression secondary to hallucinations and delusions. This can be mistaken for a panic attack, but an informant history and an examination of the mental state will usually reveal the underlying cause. In an elderly individual, such a presentation should be regarded as delirium until proved otherwise, particularly if the patient is also cognitively impaired and physically ill (see Chapter 6)

Schizophrenia

Elderly individuals with functional psychoses sometimes find their hallucinatory experiences and imagined persecutions very frightening and upsetting, but this is unlikely to cause any diagnostic difficulty. Sometimes the patient's complaints need cross-checking: is this eccentric, isolated old man deluded, or is it true that children are breaking into his flat to taunt him?

Physical illness

As we have seen, physical illness is strongly associated with anxiety and depression in old age: as a cause, as a consequence and as a mimic of these disorders. The clinical task, therefore, is to carefully delineate the physical and psychological problems that are present, and the nature and extent of any relationship between them. A physical examination, ECG and routine screening laboratory investigations will pick up most of the more common primary physical causes of neurotic symptoms in elderly patients, such as myocardial infarct, cardiac arrythmia, left ventricular failure, COPD, endocrine and metabolic disorders, anaemia and vitamin deficiencies. If the patient is or has been a smoker, a chest X-ray is also useful to rule out occult bronchial carcinoma. Symptoms of anxiety may also be secondary to prescribed medications (hypoglycaemics, corticosteroids, sympathomimetics, dopamine agonists, SSRIs), or to drug withdrawal. If this routine physical screen draws a blank, who should proceed to more detailed investigations or specialist referral? One should be more suspicious of a primary cause for neurotic symptoms in old age if they appear in individuals without any past psychiatric history, and without any clear external cause such as an adverse life event or ongoing difficulties. Neurotic symptoms with a primary physical cause usually respond to treatment of the underlying disorder, but may need managing in their own right if the illness has been severe or prolonged.

Sleep disorders

At all ages, depression and anxiety are the commonest causes of disturbed sleep, and need to be considered in any patient who presents with this problem. Other causes of sleep disturbance in elderly patients include insomnia due to pain and physical disability, periodic leg movements syndrome and restless legs syndrome, and sleep apnoea. Sudden changes of environment, such as hospitalization or institutionalization, usually result in at least a transient insomnia.

Some specific neurotic disorders

Generalized anxiety (GAD)

GAD is characterized by persistent anxious mood accompanied by motor tension, autonomic symptoms, apprehensiveness and hypervigilance. Prevalence estimates of GAD in elderly populations range from about 1 to 5%. It has a chronic fluctuating course, and is frequently co-morbid with depression in old age. A significant proportion of elderly cases appear to be of late onset, associated with functional limitations due to physical disability. GAD is also a response to severe apoplectic health events such as myocardial infarct and stroke; follow-up studies indicate that in many cases this anxiety becomes a chronic problem, associated with poor functional outcomes.

Phobic disorders

Phobias are defined as the persistent and irrational fear of an object, activity or situation resulting in a compelling desire to avoid the phobic stimulus. Phobic disorders are the most common anxiety disorders in the elderly, with one-month prevalence rates of 5–10%. While many of these phobic disorders are of long standing, a significant proportion of agoraphobias in old age are of late onset, often in response to a traumatic event such as an episode of physical illness or a fall.

Panic disorder

Panic disorder is characterized by recurrent attacks of intense fear, accompanied by severe somatic anxiety symptoms. Little is known about panic disorder in old age, but evidence from case reports, volunteer samples and non-psychiatric populations suggest that its frequency declines with increasing age, and that late-onset cases are symptomatically less severe than those whose disorder started earlier in life.

Obsessive–compulsive disorder (OCD)

OCD is characterized by obsessive thoughts and/or compulsive acts which are a significant source of distress, or interfere with social functioning. Although OCD is currently classified as one of the anxiety disorders, it is rather different from them in being a relatively stable diagnosis over time, and having a more substantial genetic component in its aetiology. The compulsive behaviours of OCD are similar to the stereotypes seen in disorders such as Tourette's syndrome and Sydenham's chorea. OCD tends to appear in young adulthood, and it is unusual for first onset to occur after the age of 50 years. However, it is a chronic and recurrent disorder and a significant proportion of cases may present to services for the first time in old age. The late onset of obsessional symptoms may form part of a primary affective disorder, or there may be an organic cause such as dementia or a space-occupying lesion affecting the frontal lobes. The anxious orderliness associated with the onset of dementia tends not to be associated with the tension that is typical of OCD.

Post-traumatic stress disorder (PTSD)

PTSD occurs following exposure to an extreme stressor, and the syndrome includes re-experiencing the trauma, avoidance, numbing and increased arousal. Little is known about PTSD in the elderly population, but the disorder can persist for many years, sometimes manifesting itself for the first time in old age.

Somatoform disorders

Somatoform disorders in late life are still poorly understood. Very few individuals of any age meet the exacting diagnostic criteria of systems such as DSM-III or

DSM-IV, which require the presence of large numbers of uncommon medically unexplained symptoms. Conditions such as ICD-10 neurasthenia, fibromyalgia and fatigue syndromes are more prevalent in both community and clinical populations, although it is not known to what extent they are over- or under-represented in older age groups. Similarly, the life course of these disorders has not been studied systematically, but clinical experience suggests that, when severe, they can be very persistent.

By definition, somatization disorder has its onset in early adult life, so elderly patients with the condition usually come with thick notes and long histories of investigation and intervention. They may have avoided psychiatrists earlier in life, and have deeply entrenched behaviours and beliefs about their symptoms that will be difficult to challenge. The onset of genuine physical ill health in old age complicates matters still further.

In contrast to the somatizer, the hypochondriac is concerned that they might be ill, and they usually present to services looking for investigation rather than treatment. Hypochondriasis arising in old age is usually secondary to another disorder, such as depression.

Management of neurotic disorders in old age

Within health services, most neurotic disorders in elderly patients are encountered in primary care and the general hospital, and this is where they should be managed, at least in the first instance. Old-age psychiatry services are usually not resourced to provide for this group, except in the more severe and intractable cases. However, they are an important source of education and support to colleagues in other clinical and residential settings; this can be offered when it becomes apparent from referrals for specialist help that they are having difficulty identifying or dealing with certain problems. As specialist old-age liaison–consultation services are developed, there will be more opportunities to offer training and supervision to staff working in acute medical units.

Psychological approaches

Cognitive behaviour therapy (CBT)
Despite the fact that interventions such as supportive therapy and CBT are of proven efficacy for a wide range of neurotic disorders in adults, and associated with fewer adverse side effects than drug treatments, their use with elderly patients is still quite limited. Admittedly, the evidence base for their effectiveness is smaller for older than for younger adults, but it has been consistently shown that for the relatively high-functioning young-old (usually) female patient with GAD, both supportive therapy and CBT are superior to staying on a waiting list, with an average effect size of 0.55. Positive results with CBT have also been reported for elderly patients with depression, panic and phobias. Elderly patients' limited access to these forms of treatment is more likely due to the current scarcity of

resources (trained therapists) and ageism within services. Whatever resources are allocated by health services for particular psychological treatments, these should be distributed equitably across all age groups, unless there is a good evidence base to indicate that this would not be cost-effective.

CBT embraces a range of educational, cognitive and behavioural therapeutic techniques that, while theoretically distinct, are usually deployed in combination to modify the problematic thinking and behaviour that occur in neurotic disorders. The cognitive component addresses the negative thoughts, false attributions and cognitive distortions that distort the patient's perception of themselves, the world, and the future, and which underlie and drive their coping style and behaviour. The behavioural component of CBT engages more directly with these behaviours, using concepts such as conditioning, avoidance, and reinforcement derived from learning theory. A common theme underpinning both the cognitive and the behavioural elements of the therapy is the encouragement of greater self-control of thoughts, feelings, and behaviour. Both approaches require the detailed assessment of the patient, which may involve diary-keeping, and the use of standardized self-report measures such as the Beck Depression Inventory, the Automatic Thought Questionnaire and the Dysfunctional Attitude Scale. A detailed individual treatment plan is then formulated, based on the findings of the assessment. This plan will involve both sessions engaged in specific tasks with the therapist, and 'homework' to build on the progress made. In patients with anxiety symptoms, these will be addressed with psychoeducation and relaxation training.

In elderly patients, the assessment will also need to include factors such as physical ill-health and disability, sensory loss, and cognitive impairment. While none of these is a contraindication to CBT per se, they may place limits on what can be achieved, or require modifications to the standard procedures. Presumably there are some individuals, for example those with severe dysmnesia, with whom little can be achieved; however, it is not yet clear where the limits to the efficacy of CBT lie in this age group. Another issue requiring further study in older patients is the use of individual versus group CBT. Group treatment has the advantage of being more cost-effective, and it can harness useful peer-group support to improve outcomes. However, problems can arise if the group is too heterogeneous and lacks important shared experiences; careful selection and preparation of patients is important, but can be time-consuming and difficult. More task-based interventions, such as anxiety management and relaxation training, may be easier to deliver effectively in a group context.

Psychodynamic therapy

For a long time, psychoanalysts and other psychodynamically oriented psychotherapists followed Freud in his belief that 'near or above the age of 50 the elasticity of the mental processes, on which treatment depends, is as a rule lacking – old people are no longer educable …'. In the past 30 years, however, a number of authors have become interested in the psychodynamics of the ageing process, and the role of the therapist in helping those individuals who have difficulty adjusting to this. The most important theme discussed in this literature is that of loss – of health, of status, of family and friends, of sexual vigour, of life – and the various difficult and destructive ways that some individuals respond to this as they grow old. These include anxiety, depression, anger, envy, acting out, passive-aggression, and somatization, all of which are commonly encountered in the elderly patients seen by health and social care services.

How, then, should psychodynamically oriented therapists contribute to the treatment and care of elderly patients? Clearly, there will never be enough such therapists available or willing to offer individual treatment to all who might benefit, so this limited expertise needs to be deployed carefully. There may be a few particularly difficult, dangerous, and resource- intensive patients who need to be taken on for long-term individual or group therapy, but therapists will probably have the greatest impact through the education and supervision of other health professionals, all of whom need some understanding of psychodynamics, defence mechanisms, and transference issues in order to work effectively with this client group. They can also help health professionals to reflect on the dynamics that operate within their team, and between their service and other agencies in the wider world.

Drug treatments

Despite the efficacy and better safety profile of psychological interventions such as CBT, most elderly patients with anxiety are still treated with drugs. This is rather surprising, given that the evidence base is still extremely limited, and most of our practice is based on the literature on younger adults, and on clinical experience and anecdote. Rational prescribing should adhere to the following principles:

1. Thorough assessment and accurate diagnosis are the necessary foundations of any effective management plan. Too often in our modern fast-throughput health services, drug treatment is merely a convenient way of avoiding a more painstaking assessment of the patients' symptoms and circumstances.

2. Consider the available non-pharmacological alternatives, in particular cognitive-behavioural and environmental interventions. Medication is always only one part of a comprehensive plan that also includes psychological and social interventions such as CBT, patient education, lifestyle advice, bibliotherapy and supportive counselling. In the absence of compelling evidence for a particular form of treatment, patient preference and choice are important considerations.

3. 'Start low and go slow'. Many of the drugs used in the management of anxiety are less efficiently metabolized and eliminated in elderly patients.

4. Set clear goals for the treatment at the outset. These might include: symptom relief without sedation; improvement in sleep; freedom from adverse physical and cognitive side effects; and avoidance of physical dependence and drug interactions. These goals should be agreed with the patient, to facilitate discontinuation if they are not achieved.

5. Give an adequate trial of treatment. Some drugs, e.g. antidepressants, can take some weeks to have their full effect.
6. At the outset, decide how long the course of anxiolytic drug treatment will be. Many patients end up with repeat prescriptions merely because no thought has been given as to whether the drug is still needed.
7. Be aware of the possible adverse consequences of treatment, for example: unpleasant or risky side effects, drug interactions, potential for dependency and abuse, and toxicity in overdose.

Drug treatment of specific disorders

Acute anxiety reactions

An anxious response to stressful events is not uncommon at any age. In some circumstances (for example, before a medical or dental procedure) it may be appropriate to manage this with a short course of a short-acting benzodiazepine (e.g. oxazepam, lorazepam; see below), in addition to reassurance and explanation. It is likely that much of what is labelled 'agitation' in individuals with severe dementia is in fact acute anxiety, and if drug treatment is required a benzodiazepine may be safer and more effective than a neuroleptic (see Chapter 5).

Generalized anxiety disorder

At all ages, benzodiazepines are the most frequently prescribed drug in the management of GAD; in both younger and more elderly patients, the limited available evidence indicates they are better than placebo. Antidepressant drugs, such as paroxetine and venlafaxine, have also been shown to be effective anxiolytics in younger patients with GAD. Treatment with an antidepressant should always be considered in elderly GAD patients with co-morbid depressive symptoms. For a more detailed account of antidepressant treatment in this age group, see Chapter 7.

The acute phase of treatment of GAD lasts a few weeks, and the aim is resolution of symptoms. The chronic phase aims to optimize the use of medication with minimal side effects. In elderly patients, short-acting benzodiazepines should be used to avoid drug accumulation and troublesome side effects such as daytime drowsiness, cognitive impairment, ataxia, fatigue, paradoxical reactions, and respiratory depression. Patients develop tolerance to the effects of benzodiazepines, so they should not be used for long-term treatment; in these circumstances, an anxiolytic antidepressant or buspirone is preferable. However, because of the delayed onset of action of the antidepressants and buspirone, initial short-term treatment with a benzodiazepine may be necessary. Bear in mind that benzodiazepines may cause rebound anxiety on dose reduction or withdrawal.

Panic disorder

The lack of evidence regarding treatment of panic disorder in the elderly is probably a consequence of its relative rarity in this population. Selective serotonin reuptake inhibitors (SSRIs) are currently the drugs of first choice for panic attacks and panic disorder in younger adults. Some patients with panic disorder experience feelings of increased anxiety when beginning treatment with an SSRI. For that reason, the initial dose should be lower than that usually prescribed to patients with depression. Panic does not respond to SSRI treatment for at least four weeks, and a full response may take 8 to 12 weeks. The initial phase of treatment may be covered by the addition of a short course of a short-acting benzodiazepine.

Obsessive-compulsive disorder (OCD)

OCD is usually treated with a combination of drug treatment and cognitive-behavioural therapy. Clomipramine is the most extensively studied treatment for OCD, but significant anticholinergic and antihistaminic side effects limit its usefulness in elderly patients. In this age group, the drug of first choice would be one of the SSRIs. The effective dose for the treatment of OCD with SSRIs tends to be higher than that required for depression, and the time taken to respond is typically much longer, at about 18 weeks. Long-term therapy is required, as discontinuation of medication usually leads to relapse. Evidence for the use of other drugs in OCD is very limited, although augmentation of SSRI treatment with either buspirone or lithium may be effective. Drug treatment appears to be more effective for obsessional thoughts than for compulsive behaviours.

Phobic disorders

As in younger patients, cognitive-behavioural therapy is the treatment of choice for phobic disorders in old age, and drugs have a relatively minor role to play.

Post-traumatic stress disorder

SSRIs such as paroxetine and sertraline have been shown to be of benefit in the treatment of PTSD in younger adults.

Somatoform disorders

There are no studies of any form of treatment in elderly patients. In younger adults, antidepressants do not appear to be effective in chronic fatigue, but they may help patients with fibromyalgia and chronic pain.

B. Personality disorders

Introduction

Personality and its disorders in old age have been very little studied, either in clinical groups or in the general population. It is commonly supposed that personality changes with age, but most models of personality development would in fact predict a stable construct after the formative influences of early life have had their effect. The limited evidence from a few longitudinal studies supports the notion that personality remains relatively stable throughout adult life, apart perhaps from some increase in introversion with age. It may be that the impression of change given by cross-sectional studies is due to cohort effects. That is, the personalities and attitudes of today's elderly people were formed at a very different time and in a very different culture from today's young adults.

What may change with age is not so much one's particular cluster of personality traits, but the specific advantages and vulnerabilities they may confer at different times of life. Indeed, personality and coping styles are likely to be important factors (along with others, such as health, income, education) determining how an individual adjusts to the various challenges of growing up and growing old. How one should adapt to old age, and just what constitutes 'successful ageing' are questions that tend to receive rather value-laden responses from writers and researchers, with much debate revolving around whether it is more appropriate to remain active, or to disengage from the world and its cares. In general, it appears that a good quality of life in old age is associated with maintaining one's interests and social networks, but there is still much we do not know about personality and adjustment to ageing, and it is likely that individuals will differ considerably in what kind of coping strategies and psychological defences work best for them. There are some coping styles that do appear to be associated with poor adjustment to old age, however. In particular, rigid and narcissistic individuals have great difficulty in accepting the limitations, disappointments and petty humiliations of ageing, and may respond by either angrily demanding or refusing the support of others. In the context of depression, such traits are an important risk factor for self-harm and suicide in old age.

Personality disorders are characterized by pervasive, enduring, extreme, and inflexible patterns of behaviour in response to a wide range of personal and social situations. They are usually, but not always, associated with subjective distress and impairment of functioning. In the modern psychiatric classifications, specific categories of personality disorder are described and defined (see Table 9.2); in DSM-IV these are grouped into three clusters in a separate axis (Axis II) from the other psychiatric disorders (Axis I). This approach has brought a degree of clarity and rigour to a complex field, but there are a number of important shortcomings. As with the neurotic disorders, the imposition of categorical diagnoses onto what are essentially dimensional constructs leads to problems such as how to classify individuals who do not fully meet diagnostic criteria for one or more disorders but who are nevertheless clearly disturbed. The relationship between Axis I and Axis II disorders is not always clear; for example, where does chronic anxiety belong? With regard to older patients, an important problem is that the diagnostic criteria do not take any account of age-related issues that may influence the presentation of personality disorder, such as physical illness or disability; cognitive impairment; and changes in social role and functioning (e.g. retirement, lack of social support). As a result, some personality disorders may be inappropriately over- or under-diagnosed in this age group. Another problem with older patients is that it may be difficult to obtain a history of problems dating back to childhood and early adulthood.

There have as yet been no longitudinal studies that have followed patients with the full range of personality disorders into old age, but cross-sectional

Table 9.2 Current classifications of personality disorders.

ICD-10	DSM-IV
ORGANIC MENTAL DISORDERS	
F07: ***Personality and behavioural disorders due to brain disease, damage and dysfunction***	
.0: Organic personality disorder	
.1: Postencephalitic syndrome	
.2: Postconcussional syndrome	
.4: Other	
.5: Unspecified	
DISORDERS OF ADULT PERSONALITY AND BEHAVIOUR	AXIS II: PERSONALITY DISORDERS
F60: ***Specific personality disorders***	*Cluster A*
.0: Paranoid	Paranoid
.1: Schizoid	Schizoid
.2: Dissocial	Schizotypal
.3: Emotionally unstable	
.30: Impulsive type	*Cluster B*
.31: Borderline type	Antisocial
.4: Histrionic	Borderline
.5: Anankastic	Histrionic
.6: Anxious (avoidant)	Narcissistic
.7: Dependent	
.8: Other specific personality disorders	
.9: Personality disorder, unspecified	*Cluster C*
	Avoidant Dependent
F61: *Mixed and other personality disorders*	Obsessive–compulsive
.0: Mixed personality disorders	
.1: Troublesome personality changes	
F62: ***Enduring personality changes, not attributable to brain damage and disease***	
.0: After catastrophic experience	
.1: After psychiatric illness	
.2: Other	
.3: Unspecified	

studies using standardized questionnaires and classifications show a different ent profile of personality disorders at different ages. In younger patients, the most prevalent DSM Axis II disorders are antisocial, borderline and passive-aggressive, whereas in older patients paranoid, schizoid and anankastic disorders are more common. It has been proposed that Axis II disorders may divide into those that are 'immature' (mostly Cluster B) and those that are 'mature' (mostly Cluster A). The mature disorders tend to be more stable with increasing age, whereas the immature disorders appear to ameliorate over time. Long-term follow-up studies of antisocial and borderline personality support this maturation hypothesis. A key element of this maturation may be a reduction in impulsivity and aggression with age, as the disorders of young adulthood are all characterized by lability of affect and behaviour. Surveys of various clinical populations agree that DSM personality disorders become less common with age. This may be because the immature disorders are declining, but it is also possible that current diagnostic systems are not very good at capturing personality disorder as it is manifest in old age.

Personality disorder and psychiatric disorder

Both dysfunctional personality traits and more severe personality disorders are known to be associated with Axis I psychiatric disorders, but the nature of this relationship is complex and multifactorial. There are of course problems with accurately determining premorbid personality during and after an episode of psychiatric disorder, but research to date does indicate that depressed and anxious patients have higher rates of premorbid personality dysfunction. This is more pronounced in younger than older patients, with older patients more likely to have Cluster C (anxious–fearful) criteria. Although evidence is limited, there are indications that it is those elderly patients with an onset of depression in early life that show the highest rates of premorbid personality dysfunction.

With regard to late-onset schizophrenia, this is associated with higher rates of Cluster A personality disorders, although it is sometimes difficult in practice to distinguish between these disorders and the prodromal phase of schizophrenia (see Chapter 8).

An issue of some clinical importance is the extent to which co-morbid personality dysfunction influences the outcome of an episode of psychiatric disorder. Evidence is limited, suggesting that while there may not be an effect on short-term outcome, rates of relapse and service use in the longer term are more frequent. Dependent traits may be associated with more chronic forms of depression. Specific adverse outcomes, such as deliberate self-harm and suicide, have been shown to be associated with Cluster C traits in late life.

Personality and organic brain disorders

This is another challenge to the current classifications and methods of assessment. Behaviour change in the context of disorders such as dementia or stroke is well-recognized, particularly if the frontal lobes are involved, and recognizing and managing this is an important part of the care of these patients. However, it is often not clear to what extent these changes in behaviour are secondary to cognitive impairment, or to the coarsening or exaggeration of premorbid personality traits. The assessment of personality in the context of cognitive impairment is of course very difficult, and usually requires informants; their judgements, however, have been found to be unreliable.

Management of personality disorders in old age

Personality disorders at all ages have traditionally been deemed to be untreatable, with management consisting of structural and environmental interventions to limit their adverse consequences. However, an evidence base is beginning to develop, at least in younger adults, for the efficacy of some forms of psychological intervention in these disorders, notably psychodynamic and cognitive therapies (see above). Unfortunately, most of the trials to date have been in patients with borderline and antisocial personality disorders, not in the Cluster A and C conditions more commonly encountered in elderly patients. There is as yet no evidence to support the use of drug treatments for personality disorders in elderly patients; in the individual case, the presence or absence of a co-morbid Axis I disorder would be the best guide to appropriate pharmacotherapy.

In the absence of evidence, what is to be done? There should be careful assessment, diagnosis and treatment of any underlying Axis I disorders. What on first acquaintance appear to be dysfunctional personality traits may in fact turn out to be symptoms of a chronic and inadequately treated affective disorder. The role, if any, of organic brain disease also needs to be determined. Physical illness and disability need to be assessed and their management optimized. At this point there needs to be a realistic setting of goals, agreed if possible with the patient and their family. Depending upon what these goals are, a number of interventions may then be tried, such as cognitive-behavioural strategies to target specific behaviours (for example, deliberate self-harm or substance abuse); grief work; life review; and environmental adaptations up to and including institutionalization to counter isolation and self-neglect.

FURTHER READING

Article

Flint, A. (2005). Generalised anxiety disorder in elderly patients: epidemiology, diagnosis and treatment options. *Drugs and Aging,* **22**, 101–114.
Good overview from a leading expert.

Book

Goldberg, D. and Huxley, P. (1992). *Common Mental Disorders: a Biopyschosocial Model.* London: Routledge.
An important and influential book which outlines the nature, significance and treatability of neurotic disorders in clear, straightforward prose.

10

Substance abuse and iatrogenesis in late life

Introduction

Substance abuse in the elderly is usually under-recognized as a problem and neglected as a significant risk factor in the development of some mental disorders in this population. Research in this area is sparse.

Alcohol abuse is more prevalent than other substance abuse in the elderly, but alcohol use disorders had not had adequate attention in their recognition and management.

There is a complex relationship between alcohol consumption and the physical and mental health of the elderly, whose age-related physiological function alterations will change this relationship as compared with young adults. The social environments of the elderly are generally different from those of the young and tend to change over time, which will have an impact upon their psychosocial stability and patterns of alcohol use.

Health professionals working with the elderly require special alertness in their clinical work so as not to miss identifying these syndromes and therefore providing prompt and effective assistance to elderly who have 'hidden' alcohol use or substance use disorders.

Alcohol use disorders

Prevalence

There are very few well-constructed epidemiological studies that have examined alcohol use and abuse among representative aged populations. Those that are available have methodological issues involving definitions, measurements and confounding factors that require attention when interpreting the data relevant to older persons.

Most studies express self-reports in a number of drinks or drinking days or number of drinks per day. In the quantity/frequency approach, subjects are asked to report what they drink on different days using a 'standard drink' as a reference. The results are then expressed as average number of drinks (or units) per day, per week, and so on. However, this approach will not account for some patterns of drinking such as binge drinking, past heavy consumption with current lower consumption or cumulative alcohol consumption over a lifetime.

In Australia a standard drink is defined as 10 g of alcohol, which is found in 375 ml of light beer or 285 ml of regular strength beer, 30 ml of spirits, 90–120 ml of wine. European studies use 8 g as a standard drink, while in the USA it is 0.5 ounces (13 g) of alcohol, which is equivalent to 1.5 ounces (45 ml) of spirits, 5 ounces (150 ml) of wine and 12 ounces (360 ml) of beer.

In the USA, light to moderate drinking is 1–2 drinks per day, whereas in the Rotterdam Health Study, 1–3 drinks per week is the benchmark; 1–6 drinks in the Cardiovascular Health Study.

Community surveys report a range of alcohol abuse prevalence rates from 1% (Liverpool, UK), 27% of men (Newcastle-upon-Tyne, UK) to 22% of men and 2% of women in a US study. In treatment settings the alcohol abuse prevalence rate ranges from a low of 6.5% (Nottingham, UK), 7.5% (Adelaide, Australia) of psychogeriatric in-patients to a high of 21% in a general hospital in-patient study from Baltimore, USA.

However, most community studies do report a decline in alcohol consumption with increasing age in cross-sectional studies. Whether this is due to a true decrease or whether it reflects differences in cohort effects, increased physiological effects per drink, medical problems which impact on accessibility and/or desirability of alcohol, aspects of the changing social and domestic lifestyle of the elderly, or simply the likelihood that heavy drinkers die young, is quite opaque.

Metabolism of alcohol in late life

With increasing age, physiological changes will alter the metabolism of all substances including alcohol. Changes in absorption, plasma binding and renal excretion and decreased body water all lead to higher blood alcohol concentrations. Such physiological changes together with altered metabolism are likely to result in the occurrence of more damage for the same level of intake compared with younger people. Associated with this are the altered effects of alcohol in the elderly such as increased functional impairment with the same blood levels, decreased euphoric effects, and decreased capacity to develop tolerance. Alcohol also will aggravate medical and psychiatric diseases and disorders, increase cognitive impairment and reduce sensory and motor capacity.

Such increases in the damaging effects of alcohol use in the elderly would need to be factored in when assessing the alcohol intake of older adults.

Health-related effects of excessive consumption of alcohol in the elderly

While the major effects of excess alcohol consumption overlaps that of the younger adult, there are special considerations applying to the elderly. Heavy intake (five or more drinks daily) is associated with a quadrupled risk of developing cognitive impairment. A problem drinking history increases the risk of depression, psychiatric illnesses and memory problems quite substantially.

While only 20% of studies report harm associated with increased alcohol exposure, the physician should be alerted to individuals whose increased alcohol intake may be associated with (if not causal for) risk of falls and fractures, decreased functional ability, driving impairment, drug interaction and delirium.

Although heavy alcohol consumption is an established risk in the development of dementia, recent population studies including the Rotterdam Study, the Copenhagen City Heart Study and the Cardiovascular Health Study have suggested, however, that light to moderate drinking (1–3 drinks per day: Rotterdam Study; 1–6 drinks per day: Cardiovascular Health Study) is associated with a lower risk for dementia. The Copenhagen City Heart Study showed no relationship between alcohol intake and the risk of dementia. Exclusive wine drinkers seem to have a lower risk of developing dementia. Such a conclusion was also reached in a Stockholm Study.

The relationship between alcohol dependence and suicide in a Swedish Study revealed that a history of alcohol dependence was observed in 35% of elderly men and 18% of elderly women who died by suicide. On the other hand, in the control group 2% of men and 1% of women had alcohol dependence or misuse. The odds ratio was calculated to be 18-fold in men with an alcohol disorder and 9.5-fold in women. Alcohol use disorder is an independent risk factor for predicting suicide in the elderly and is associated with non-violent methods in the final act.

Late-onset alcoholism

A significant proportion of alcohol abusers take up heavy drinking in old age. This leads to the concept of 'late-onset alcoholism'. This term refers to those whose previous 'normal' drinking habits become heavy and to previous non-drinkers who develop alcohol abuse in late life.

The physical, mental and environmental effects of ageing seem to be related to this change from normal to pathological alcohol intake. Reactive life factors such as bereavement, retirement, loneliness, physical infirmity and relationship stress are indicators of risk.

This concept, however, is not universally accepted, as most elderly people do not drink excessively despite the 'stresses of ageing', and not all late-onset drinkers attribute such stresses as reasons for their drinking.

It is likely that a small group of elderly people may develop drinking problems for the first time in late life when they adversely react to negative life events such as bereavement and retirement. The possibility of better prognosis and response to intervention in restoring their life and psychological balance should lead to some level of optimism when these elderly patients are identified.

Management of alcohol problems in the elderly

The first step in management begins with identification of the problem. Some special and personal changes provide suggestive pointers which should raise the clinician's suspicions. Self-neglect is associated with cognitive decline; evidence of poor nutrition; unexplained falls, accidents, injuries; unstable and poorly controlled physical illness (diabetes, hypertension); failure to keep appointments and poor compliance with treatment; increasing conflict with family members; the persistence of gastrointestinal problems; unexplained delirium during hospitalization for medical treatment are all possible pointers to the presence of alcohol abuse.

When late-life alcohol abuse is suspected, a detailed history of alcohol intake needs to be checked with family members and a visit to the home should be scheduled. During this visit there should be inspection to check for stacks of empty bottles in the back garden or the rubbish bins, any stock of alcohol in cupboards and pantries and any evidence of neglect of the home should be noted.

Should detoxification be required, this must be done in hospital, particularly if the patient is at risk of life-threatening sequelae of intoxication, accidental events or severe risk to existing medical illness. During detoxification it will be necessary to be alert for the withdrawal symptoms of *delirium tremens* including tremor, insomnia, sweating, nausea or vomiting, transient frightening visual, auditory or tactile hallucinations, psychomotor hyperactivity, severe anxiety and fear, autonomic hyperactivity and withdrawal seizures.

Time-limited use of short-acting benzodiazepines can be useful in treatment of symptoms of alcohol withdrawal. Thiamine (both intravenous and oral) with other vitamin supplements is always useful, as most alcohol abusers are nutritionally impaired. The use of novel antipsychotics with sedating properties in low doses may be required to manage frightening hallucinations, although these drugs can lower the fit threshold. General supportive care aimed towards restoration of physiological and psychological balance should be undertaken during detoxification.

After detoxification, the management will include a thorough assessment of both the physical and psychosocial status of the patient. In particular, the repertoire of psychological and personality strengths and resilience in the history of the patient should be utilized. Such factors will be useful tools to be deployed in psychotherapeutic interventions to follow. The strengths, extent and availability of family support will also be assessed. Identifying and treating medical and psychiatric co-morbidity must be undertaken thoroughly. Depression, hypertension, and cardiovascular diseases, painful conditions such as arthritis, late-onset (type II) diabetes will all need to be investigated and treated energetically, as these frequently contribute to both the general well-being of the patient, and management can remove some of the contributing effects of disability secondary to alcohol over-use.

Psychotherapeutic interventions using such strategies as cognitive behavioural therapy, interpersonal psychotherapy, marital/family therapy as indicated, will be the mainstay of resolving basic underlying drivers in the patient's motivation to continue alcohol abuse.

The adjunctive contribution of spiritual support in patients who have a past history of spiritual activities, or who wish to embark on a new spiritual direction, should always be included in a holistic programme management. As in all areas of old-age psychiatry, the multidisciplinary model involving all health care professionals – physiotherapy, occupational therapy, nursing, dietician, podiatrist, speech pathologist – in the care of these patients will contribute to the success of treatment, as such professionals add to the quality of life and thus add positive meaning to counter the urge to return to (ab)using alcohol.

Outcome

Although existing studies generally tend to be pessimistic regarding interventions, with about 1 in 7 having good outcomes, it is to be noted that those who did continue in treatment programmes were more likely to be successful. These are late-onset drinkers who are often socially isolated, widowed and highly motivated. An expansion of social networks was associated with improvement and with completion of therapy. Keeping the patient in treatment programmes by enhancing their expectations and motivations, thus providing an expanded social network and support, may be necessary ingredients for a better outcome.

Other substance abuse disorders and iatrogenesis

Illicit substances

Members of the current generation of elderly are not much given to the abuse of illicit substances available to younger adults. However, as the 'baby boomers' start to attain the status of older persons by 2010, there will be an increasing number whose use of illicit substances in their youth will either continue or resume in old age. This 'baby boomer' generation will bring with them new challenges and open up new varieties of mental health problem, currently not much encountered in routine old-age psychiatry practice.

At this stage, health professionals should prepare themselves to be vigilant in identifying those who may use illicit drugs either as a lifestyle habit or who abuse them as a substitute for psychosocial support in their old age.

Prescribed medications – iatrogenesis

A more serious current problem in substance abuse is that of prescribed dependency-promoting medications.

The entry of benzodiazepines into the medical world was an initial boon as this displaced the barbiturate dependence problem which was quite serious in the 1950s and 1960s. Members of the current generation of older people sometimes were switched from barbiturates to benzodiazepines for the treatment of anxiety and insomnia while others had benzodiazepine drugs initiated *de novo* and continued to receive prescriptions for these drugs for many years thereafter. Some have continued on the same dosage into their old age with little harm. However, dependence has occurred in some people who, after entering old age, began to use benzodiazepines to manage their emotional and psychological distress as well as for their depression and early cognitive change, while others have continued an earlier pattern of dependence or abuse into their later years. Such dependence has serious health consequences which may include multiple falls and fractures with resulting disability and even death. Many studies have identified the role of benzodiazepine hypnotics (even in the non-dependent elderly) as a major risk factor in falls and fractures, especially in residential care. Excessive sedation can encourage immobility and may increase the risk of hypostatic pneumonia, aggravate joint pathology and reduce exposure to sunlight with resistant vitamin deficiencies and consequent bone disorders. The quality of life impacts of the over-use of benzodiazepines among old people are of major medical and ethical concern.

Current best practice advice is that if benzodiazepines are indicated at all for older adults, they must be used in the lowest possible dose for the shortest period of time and be reviewed regularly to see if the dosage can be reduced or be ceased altogether.

Health professionals working in residential care should be always alert to the harmful effects of benzodiazepine over-use and exercise due care in preventing such problems from developing. The use of benzodiazepines for 'behavioural control' is at best inappropriate and at worst may represent professional misconduct. Virtually all elderly people who experience problems of benzodiazepine toxicity, withdrawal symptoms or other adverse effects started to take them on medical advice. Despite the fact that the elderly are the most vulnerable members of the population to the adverse effects of benzodiazepine use, despite falling rates of prescription they continue to be more likely to be prescribed these drugs than are younger adults. Prevention is better than cure, and in this case the solution to the problem lies in medical practitioners initiating the prescription of these drugs less often and less readily to elderly patients.

Conclusion

Professional health care workers who see older adults should always be alert to the misuse and abuse of alcohol and prescribed substances as well as illicit substances. The comprehensive management of a biopsychosocial spiritual approach will be necessary to assist old people who misuse and abuse such substances. Alertness in identifying pointers to substance misuse and abuse requires constant vigilance on the part of all of us who care for the elderly. A sensitive and caring questioning of the older patient in these areas is necessary and should always be part of history taking and examination, as well as a necessary component of any home visits.

Multidisciplinary and multimodal treatments should be applied energetically and optimistically to ensure the best possible and improved quality of life. In the endeavour to assist old people affected by substance abuse, the professional's strongest ally will usually be the patient's family.

FURTHER READING

Articles

Ganguli, M., Vanderbilt, J., Saxton, J. A., Shen, C. and Dodge H. H. (2005). Alcohol consumption and cognitive function in late life. *Neurology,* **65**, 1210–1217.
Highlights the potential for harm associated with late-life alcohol abuse.

Graham, K., Carver V. and Brett, P. J. (1996). Alcohol and drug use by older women: result of a national survey. *Canadian Journal of Ageing,* **14**, 769–791.
A good study giving plausible prevalence figures.

Graham, K., *et al.* (1996). Addictive behaviour in older adults. *Addictive Behaviour,* **21**, 331–348.
An account of the phenomenon of addiction in late life with regard to prescribed substances as well as licit and illicit drugs of abuse.

Patterson, T. L. and Jeste, D. V. (1999). The potential impact of Baby-Boomer generation on substance abuse amongst elderly persons. *Psychiatric Services,* **50**, 1184–1188.
Highlights the possible effects of the maturation of the postwar generation on substance abuse patterns.

Rigler, S. K. (2000). Alcoholism in the elderly. *American Family Physician,* **61**, 1710–1766.
Focuses on the more severe end of the alcohol abuse spectrum in late life.

Ticehurst, S. (1990). Alcohol in the elderly. *Australian and New Zealand Journal of Psychiatry,* **24**, 252–260.
This clear and thorough article is still pertinent 20 years after it was written.

Whelan, G. (2003). Alcohol: a much neglected risk factor in elderly mental disorders. *Current Opinion in Psychiatry,* **1**, 609–614.
Evidence-based overview which is well written.

Book chapter

Gambert, S. and Albriecht II, C. (2005). The elderly. In J. L. Lewinson, P. Ruiz, R. Millman and J. G. Langrod, (Eds.) *Substance Abuse: a Comprehensive Textbook, 4th edition* (pp. 1038–1048). Philadelphia, PA: Lippincott Williams and Wilkins.
Another useful source of information on the topic of substance abuse in late life.

11

Services for older patients with psychiatric disorders

Brief historical notes

The emergence of dedicated services for older people with mental disorders is a fairly recent phenomenon in health services around the world. Until the 1950s, elderly people with severe mental disorders were treated and housed in large mental hospitals located away from the general community.

In the 1950s, important research into the mental disorders of late life began in the UK. This work highlighted the fact that these disorders are important entities deserving special attention. Reports of a series of scandals stirred policy makers to consider new management models. This, in conjunction with a more positive attitude towards the elderly derived from the research of Roth, Kiloh, Kay, Blessed, Bergman, Corsellis, Post and others combined to lead to a more enlightened approach. In the USA, Butler at the Institute of Mental Health led research in human ageing, whilst in 1959 the World Health Organization convened the first meeting of its expert committee on the mental health of the aged, which was followed in 1965 by the World Psychiatric Association (WPA) holding a Conference on 'Mental Disorders in the Aged'.

From the 1960s in Britain and North America, a process of development of special attention towards the mentally disordered elderly, focused on moving those with serious mental illnesses out of the large mental hospitals into community settings. By the 1980s, especially in the UK, emerging specialist services for old people came into being, underpinned by the principles of comprehensive old-age psychiatry services – flexibility, responsiveness, availability, un-hierarchical use of staff, domiciliary assessment, and willingness to collaborate with other services and agencies.

This British model was championed by Tom Arie, who, through the British Council courses in psychogeriatrics, promulgated it to other parts of the world including Canada, Australia, Continental Europe, Scandinavia, South Africa and Hong Kong. Many of the old-age psychiatry services in developed countries around the world adapted this 'Arie Model' to suit local conditions.

International consensus model on organizations of care

The influence of the British leaders in the early development of psychogeriatric services (Arie, Pitt, Post, Jolley) led to the establishment of services to old people which included comprehensive assessment (preferably at the person's locale), and served the population of potential patients in a local community.

Central to this is the multidisciplinary psychogeriatric team with a consultant psychiatrist, committed to old people, leading such a team which includes nurses, social workers, occupational therapists, psychologists (clinical and/or neuropsychologists) and other health professionals such as physiotherapists, podiatrists, dietiaians, music therapists and pharmacists according to local circumstances.

As differing models of service delivery evolved, especially in the UK, USA, Australia and Continental Europe by the mid-1990s, an international consensus was seen to be necessary to establish what could be considered as core international best practice.

To achieve this, the late Jean Wertheimer of Lausanne, Switzerland, as the Chair of the World Psychiatric Association Section of Geriatric Psychiatry, took the initiative in 1997 in organizing a very successful Consensus Conference. Thus a Consensus Statement, with the imprimatur of the WPA and WHO, with the participation of related international bodies such as IPA and other non-government organizations, was prepared and published. This document provides the fundamental generic model of best practice in the organization of care in psychogeriatric services delivery (see further reading section below).

Specific principles of best practice in this consensus document can be referred to as the CARITAS principles. CARITAS is the Latin word for love and care, which underpins the attitude behind the use of this acronym.

Quality care for older persons with mental health problems should be:

Comprehensive
Accessible
Responsive
Individualized
Transdisciplinary
Accountable
Systemic (seamless)

- A *comprehensive* service should take into account all aspects of the patient's physical, psychological and social needs and wishes and be patient-centred.
- An *accessible* service is user-friendly and readily available, minimizing the geographical, cultural, financial, political and linguistic obstacles to obtaining care.
- A *responsive* service is one that listens to and understands the problems brought to its attention and acts promptly and appropriately.
- An *individualized* service focuses on each person with a mental health problem in his or her family and community context. The planning of care must be tailored for and acceptable to the individual and family, and should aim wherever possible to maintain and support the person with in their home environment.
- A *transdisciplinary* approach goes beyond traditional professional boundaries to optimize the contributions of people with a range of personal and

professional skills. Such an approach also facilitates collaboration with voluntary and other agencies to provide a comprehensive range of community oriented services.

- An *accountable* service is one that accepts responsibility for assuring the quality of the service it delivers and monitors this in partnership with patients and their families. Such a service must be ethically and culturally sensitive.
- A *systemic* (seamless) approach flexibly integrates all available services to ensure continuity of care and coordinates all levels of service providers including local, provincial and national governments and community organizations.

The transdisciplinary principle needs further explanation. In less developed countries, with few professional disciplines beyond doctor and nurse, the concepts of multidisciplinary and interdisciplinary can be difficult to apply. Our Zimbabwean colleague, Dr Juliet Dube-Ddebele suggested, and the Consensus Group agreed, that the concept principle of transdisciplinary – which has the core value of transcending disciplinary boundaries to be inclusive of all available skills from professional, lay and voluntary groups – should be promoted instead of the traditional multidisciplinary or interdisciplinary principles so valued in more developed countries.

The multidisciplinary team

An essential feature of psychogeriatric care is the multidisciplinary team which works in a transdisciplinary manner. Although the old-age psychiatrist is the team leader, every attempt is made to operate in a non-hierarchical, mutually respectful and collaborative way having the welfare and quality of life of older people as a committed shared value.

Transcending disciplinary barriers can be difficult in some situations. A functional team will put such difficulties as a secondary consideration to the high priority of patient-focused decision-making.

The overlap of discipline-related skills will benefit the patient by the enhancement of practical application of discipline-specific skills. For example, the nurse may apply physiotherapy and occupational therapy skills learned from them so that out-of-hours application of their therapeutic interventions may be continued. Knowledge and skills of good nursing practice will enhance that of the therapists during therapy activities.

Residential care

Whilst the primary goal is to keep the older person living at home for as long as possible, residential care is a necessary option for those whose physical, mental health and well-being are best served in the residential care environment.

The quality of residential care applies to all aspects of the residential environment.

Design of the physical, built environment should be homely, conducive to privacy, visually pleasing and provide a sense of cheerful comfort. Light and space indoors and outside space for gentle exercise, gardens for visual and olfactory pleasure should be available. The relationship of spatial areas, colours of walls and floors should be simple, safe and orientating. The use of both easily recognized symbols and words on signage assist in orientation. Furnishings should be safe, taking into account physical disability as well as being comfortable and practical and, where possible, consistent with the period of the older peoples' life in their design. The kitchen should be open to the common space to allow for visual, auditory and olfactory contact with the residents as well as being available to those who can use their retained food preparation skills under supervision.

The television should not be used as a 'baby-sitting' device, but utilized positively for stimulating the cognitive function of residents. Music of each resident's preference in both public and private areas will provide listening pleasure, enhance reminiscences, and facilitate rhythm-related movements.

Space for leisure activities, assisted by staff members (often a recreational therapist), will enhance the enjoyment of daily life as with planned outings to places of interest, public festivals and entertainment.

Residential care, although having medical and nursing functions, should attempt to minimize the emphasis on these activities as much as possible to produce and maintain a more home-like environment.

Visitors (family, friends or volunteers) should be welcomed into the residential community and encouraged to bring the outside world into the facility to add value to residential care.

Other activities usually undertaken in the general community, such as shopping, hairdressing, tea and coffee houses, pets can be innovatively brought into the facility or available to those residents who could leave the facility safely accompanied by staff members, relatives and friends.

The wearing of uniforms by staff is a contentious issue. Where uniform is required for identification, this should be designed to minimize the 'hospital'-like atmosphere it may evoke. If identification name badges are worn, these should be in large print and strategically placed for older people to read and recognize.

Designated quiet areas for spiritual activities, contemplation, and meditation encourage those who have spiritual needs to continue to undertake their usual practices and rituals.

A deliberate emphasis on designing a sensitive and pleasing built environment not only benefits residents directly, but will engender an atmosphere in which staff will respond with more appropriate affect and attitude.

Medical care

As medical co-morbidity is common, quality energetic medical care, usually provided by visiting primary care physicians or general practitioners (GPs), should be in place. Timely access to specialist care provides support to the GPs.

Community-based assessment

The front line activity of an old-age psychiatry team is the place of domicile of patients and their families. All, or nearly all, assessment should be performed in patients' homes. The team goes to the patients rather than the patient coming to the team. Such an approach should enable the development of a more significant therapeutic alliance, shows that the patient and families are valued, removes obstacles to accessibility such as mobility difficulties, and provides the opportunity to see how life is lived in each home and provides a more practical understanding of where support may be needed.

In countries where there is a perceived legal/liability obstacle to such an approach, advocacy to alter the legal environment should be energetically pursued through the legislature.

Respite care

Carers of older persons with any disability become tired and burnt out. For those caring for people with mental disorders, this may be more so. Regular breaks (respite) for carers should be available. This can be by home-based respite where a substitute carer will replace the carer at home, thereby freeing up the carer to have respite. Removal of the patient to residential facilities for respite care is another option and may enable the carer to take lengthy (1, 2, 3 weeks or more) respite at regular intervals (2, 3, 4 times a year). Maintaining the health and well-being of the carer is a necessary part of any quality old-age psychiatry service delivery.

Information, advice and public education

The dual stigma of mental illness and ageing that is so prevalent in all countries requires constant action in de-stigmatization by old-age psychiatry services. The delivery of accurate information on both ageing and mental disorders through printed material, electronic or print media, public discussion forum, and taking any opportunity to 'sell' a positive message to the general community and the health community forms a necessary part of the work of the old-age psychiatry service. Collaboration with mental health organizations, NGOs, and carers' groups in any activity of public education will enhance what the service does by itself.

Advocacy

Elderly persons may be reluctant to speak up for themselves, participate in protest marches or undertake overt political activities to make a point or demand.

This will change as the activist-minded boomer generation will be the new cohort of the elderly.

An old-age psychiatry service with trained professionals can be the voices of their patients and families to obtain the attention of policy makers who frequently ignore this silent minority.

Equitable, accessible, affordable care services, availability of pharmaceuticals, adequate financial security, accessible and disabled-friendly transport, appropriate housing, neighbourhood resources are issues that often demand the advocacy action of the service as an entity and staff members individually. Pro-activity on behalf of the elderly has been a strong historical hallmark of early psychogeriatric services, especially in the UK. Such an example should be followed and expanded by all current and future services.

Spiritual and leisure needs

Meaningful and appropriate recreational and leisure activities contribute to quality of life of older people. Leisure which includes gentle exercise and outdoor activities as part of pleasurable activity has additional health benefits. The opportunity to express and practise spiritual aspects of their lives and lived experiences will contribute to their sense of peace as well as an effective preparation for their end of life directions. Helping them to resolve inter-personal and intra-personal conflicts through spiritual means often contribute to their dying well. Each older person's spiritual needs, expressions and practices should always be respected and honoured.

What are the necessary components of a service?

To this question, irrespective of available resources, the principle of 'surround them with care' should be central (Figure 11.1).

Resource-rich services will have more components, whereas resource-poor services will have fewer. However, rich or poor, the resources available should provide an encircling support system for the patient and family. The family, local/neighbourhood community should always be considered care components to which are added others as more resources become available. In an ideal world, the following components are considered to be the minimum acceptable:

- Community mental health teams for older persons
- In-patient assessment and treatment
- Day hospitals
- Outpatient services
- Respite care – 'in-home' or facility-based
- Continuing hospital care
- Residential care

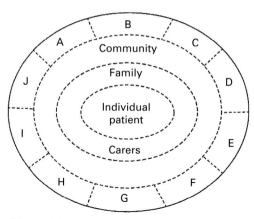

Figure 11.1 Surround them with care

- Liaison services for general and geriatric hospitals
- Primary care collaborations
- Community and social support services
- Prevention programmes
- Educational programmes for health professionals
- De-stigmatization programmes and public education and health promotion.

Innovation

Psychogeriatric services staff are usually creative and innovative people who are good problem-solvers in many practical ways. This is to be encouraged, fostered and applauded.

While advancing technology can provide effective and useful solutions (e.g. Global Positions Tracking, pressure-pad alarm systems, key-pad coded doors), there are many opportunities for staff to exercise their imagination aided by practical life experiences to resolve problems offered by patients and families. Some creative lateral thinking often produces very simple, affordable and satisfactory results.

Conclusion

The most effective quality service for older people with mental disorders is one which is patient- and family-centred; values and encourages staff; has an ethos of CARITAS towards older persons; uses resources effectively and wisely; and puts into effect despite any resource constraints, the principles as established by the WPA/WHO Consensus Statement of 1997.

FURTHER READING

Book chapters

Arie, T. (2002). The development in Britain. In J. R. M. Copeland, M. T. Abou-Saleh and D. G. Blazer, (Eds.) *Principles and Practice of Geriatric Psychiatry, 2nd edition* (pp. 9–11). Chichester: John Wiley.
Service-focused overview of the development of old-age psychiatric services in the UK.

Snowdon, J. and Arie, T. (2005). A history of psychogeriatric services. In P. Melding, B. Draper and H. Brodaty, (Eds.) *Psychogeriatric Service Delivery: an International Perspective* (pp. 3–20). Oxford: Oxford University Press.
Excellent summary of the history of our field.

Consensus statement

World Health Organization. (1997). *Consensus Statement in Organization of Care in Psychiatry of the Elderly.* WHO/MSA/MNH/97.3. Geneva: WHO.
A prescription for service creation and implementation and a guide to best practice.

12

The future of the psychiatry of old age

Introduction

An understanding of past and current trends that bear on the mental disorders of later life informs any speculation about the future. By speculating about the future, one aims to develop a successful strategy for educating future health care professionals who will care for older adults. At the same time, we aim to develop an approach that will enhance our understanding of psychiatric disorders of later life. Attempting to predict the future has always been a mug's game, yet as an exercise, it may have heuristic value. In this chapter, we summarize recent debates about how to 'go forward' with the full knowledge that the future is highly unpredictable. None the less, it is fair to say that two major issues will continue to influence the future of the psychiatry of old age (POA):

1. POA will be profoundly affected by the future of its parent discipline, that of psychiatry, and in particular the recent impact of neuroscience. In psychotherapy, the general shift towards manual- and evidenced-based short-term therapies will have a significant influence on our approach to older adults, especially those with mild cognitive impairment.
2. The second major influence will be the outcome of the recent debate about the future of geriatrics (geriatric medicine), a closely related discipline. Do we continue to provide age-based as opposed to needs-based services and sub specialties?

Historical influences

In an earlier paper written in 1994 by one of the current book's four authors (KS), speculation about the future of geriatric psychiatry began with a review of historical developments that shaped the field to that point. This included the importance of leaders in mainstream psychiatry of the 1950s and 1960s (Sir Martin Roth in Newcastle and Felix Post at the Institute of Psychiatry in London) turning their attention to the study of older adults. This had the effect of legitimizing the field of POA and attracting attention from mainstream trainees. Roth's paper on the 'Natural history of mental disorders' published in 1955 had its greatest impact by demonstrating the uniqueness of the three Ds – Dementia, Depression and Delirium. Ironically, recent work covered in other chapters has demonstrated that the independence of these syndromes is not as pronounced as originally suggested by Roth. None the less, that paper did have a profound impact on the academic and clinical interest in POA.

Service developments in the National Health Service of the UK made it easier to provide psychiatric services to the frail and cognitively impaired elderly. This in turn led pioneers in the field like Brice Pitt and Tom Arie to promote the importance of collaboration with the field of geriatric medicine. This has remained the primary specialty relationship for POA. The principles regarding the development of service delivery in the British National Health Service (NHS) for geriatrics largely informed the same approach to POA. These principles included comprehensiveness, accountability, clearly defined target populations, accessibility and flexibility of services with a strong focus on the community and the role of carers.

Several organizations have reflected and influenced the development of 'psychogeriatrics'. In Britain, the Royal College of Psychiatrists hosted the development of an interest group for Old Age Psychiatry in 1978. This small interest group of energetic and charismatic psychiatrists went on to develop a section that now has blossomed into the Faculty of Old Age Psychiatry for the Royal College of Psychiatrists and established a credible body informing health policy and principles of service delivery. The Canadian Association of Geriatric Psychiatry appears to be following the direction of the Royal College of Psychatrists by focusing on health policy, especially psychiatric consultation to nursing homes. In the USA, on the other hand, the American Association of Geriatric Psychiatry (AAGP), similarly established in 1978, became an active voice within the parent American Psychiatric Association, but focused largely on academic matters and helped to stimulate a high level of clinical research in the field of geriatric psychiatry. The success of the International Psychogeriatric Association (IPA) has also focused on the debate as to whether psychogeriatrics/POA should become more multidisciplinary and egalitarian in its approach to the mental disorders of late life, or whether it should be still largely led by the field of geriatric psychiatry with neurologists, geriatricians and other specialists as collaborators.

Clinical neuroscience

In previous speculations about the future of psychiatry and geriatrics, the fields of neurology and neuroscience have largely been neglected. However, recent literature suggests that the development of clinical neurosciences may very well represent the most powerful force for change in psychiatry and in particular for POA. This involves the increasingly close and collaborative relationship with cognitive and behavioural neurology which in turn has transformed its parent discipline of neurology over the last two decades. In 2002, Martin documented the very significant research advances in our understanding of the genetic basis of the diseases which affect the brain and central nervous system. In particular, he notes the impact of disorders such as Alzheimer's disease (AD) and Tourette's syndrome which serve as prototypes for the reasons that clinical work and research in neurology and psychiatry diverged so dramatically in the twentieth century.

Defining AD by its neuropathologic hallmarks of neuronal loss, senile plaques and neurofibrillary tangles has assigned this disorder to the neurologic category of disease, notwithstanding the fact that many of the features and symptoms of the disease are behavioural and psychiatric in nature. It is clear that despite its neurological substrate, a joint effort of neurologists and psychiatrists was necessary to understand the way diseases of the brain create an 'illness of the mind'. This conceptualization helped to blur the previously artificial categories of 'organic' and 'functional' disorders. In contrast, Gilles de la Tourette syndrome, for which there was no known neuropathological basis, remained mired in a debate about psychological versus organic causes without resolution until recent years.

Historically, the division between neurology and psychiatry became more obvious after the Second World War, when the *Archives of Neurology and Psychiatry* published in the USA was divided into two separate journals. However, this separation has become blurred as the major diseases of psychiatry such as schizophrenia and bipolar disorder are shown to be accompanied by significant changes in brain structure and function. Martin points out that since the 1960s, developments in neuropharmacology, and in particular the identification of neurotransmitter systems, has led to the development of the field known as biological psychiatry. Furthermore, developments in neuroimaging, including functional imaging techniques, MRI, PET scanning and computed tomography, have created a neuroscience base for the larger field of psychiatry. Martin reprises Winston Churchill's original characterization of the USA and Britain as two countries separated by a common language. For neurology and psychiatry, that common language is indeed neuroscience. The Nobel laureate Eric Kandel argues that psychiatry can make a contribution to brain science by 'defining for biology the mental functions that need to be studied for a meaningful and sophisticated understanding of the human mind ... The details of the relationship between the brain and mental processes – precisely how the brain gives rise to various mental processes – is understood poorly, and only in outline. The great challenge for biology and psychiatry at this point is to delineate that relationship in terms that are satisfying to both the biologist of the brain and the psychiatrist of the mind ...'.

One of the greatest stimuli for reconsidering our approach to mental disorders of late life is the relative difficulty in recruitment that has been experienced particularly in North America in the fields of geriatric medicine and to some extent geriatric psychiatry. Martin's vision for the future largely ignores the field of geriatrics and instead focuses on the need for the convergence of psychiatry, neurology and neuroscience.

In 2005, Insel and Quirion made an impassioned plea for psychiatry to have an impact on public health by helping mental disorders to be understood and treated as brain disorders. This comes from the heads of the respective national Mental Health Institutes in the USA and Canada. In the past, mental disorders immediately became the purview of neurology the moment a lesion in the brain was identified. Like Martin, they note that development of functional neuroimaging has helped to visualize patterns of abnormal regional brain activity. What follows logically from their premise is that if mental disorders are indeed primarily brain disorders, then the fundamentals of psychiatry must of necessity include neuroscience and genomics. This in turn will profoundly affect the training of future psychiatrists and may create a new clinician referred to as a 'clinical neuroscientist'. However, a concern has been raised that if psychiatry becomes a neuroscience-based disorder, we may lose the discipline's long-developed and sophisticated understanding of behaviour, emotion and the development of inter-personal skills.

Insel and Quirion note that developments in molecular genetics which identify genetic variations associated with disease will facilitate the understanding of the pathophysiology of many mental disorders and in turn reveal new targets for treatments. Genomics also provides an approach to understanding the risk of many major psychiatric disorders and in turn offers possible strategies for prevention. They highlight the recent work that shows an interaction between genes and environment, sustaining the fundamental notion that the future of psychiatry as a clinical neuroscience discipline needs to incorporate both molecular genetics, neuroscience and psychosocial factors.

Neuroimaging research involving functional magnetic resonance imaging and single photon emission computed tomography may develop biomarkers for mental disorders. For example, evidence from several sources has implicated circuitry that involves area 25 of the medial prefrontal cortex in major depressive disorder. Imaging of monoamine receptors may reveal regional abnormalities that serve as biomarkers of future diagnostic tests.

Future training in clinical neuroscience

The notion of the clinical neuroscientist was developed originally by Thomas Detre and advanced by others including Insel and Quirion. If the fundamental premise is that mental disorders, such as AD, late-life depression, paranoid disorders of late life and delirium are indeed brain disorders, then psychiatrists of the future will need to become brain scientists. Neurologists will have to shift towards a more psychosocial approach and psychiatrists towards a more fundamental understanding of neuroscience. Insel and Quirion argue that redefining psychiatry as clinical neuroscience will accelerate the integration of psychiatry with the rest of medicine and, a fortiori, this will apply to the integration of geriatric psychiatry with the rest of medicine and especially neurology and geriatric medicine. The notion that psychiatry has been separated from other medical specialties in the latter part of the twentieth century may have led to the perpetuation of the stigma that still stains individuals, families and those of us who treat people with major mental disorders. However, it may be that even beyond the stigma, the separation of mental health services from the mainstream of medicine has affected the quality of care provided to those with serious mental illness. The success of this future integration will depend on the ability of psychiatry to bring to modern neuroscience a special focus on the public health needs of those who experience mental illnesses while retaining the focus on the contribution of human experience to brain disease.

The reciprocal relationship of neurology and psychiatry is reflected in mirror papers by two of the leading researchers in the psychiatry of old age. Jeffrey Cummings, writing in 2005 on the neuropsychiatric burden of neurologic diseases in the elderly, highlighted the increasing recognition that brain dysfunction is also reflected by behavioural and affective symptoms in addition to intellectual and functional decline. Therefore, the management of brain disorders requires the involvement of psychogeriatricians and psychogeriatric services in order to manage conditions where behavioural and psychological symptoms are common and significant yet under-recognized and under-treated.

In the same issue of *International Psychogeriatrics*, John O'Brien reviewed the cognitive effects of traditional 'psychiatric disorders' such as schizophrenia, depression and bipolar disorder. O'Brien notes that in the prototypic psychiatric disorder schizophrenia, cognitive impairment has been demonstrated in a number of areas including working memory, attention, verbal and visual learning and memory, problem-solving and speed of processing. Similarly, depressed subjects have shown multiple impairments in attention, working memory, visual and verbal memory, new learning as well executive dysfunction. These cognitive deficits are not only a result of the mood disturbance (trait) but persist even after recovery from the mood disorder (state). Recent evidence has implicated the hypothalamic–pituitary–adrenal (HPA) axis and indeed in depression in older subjects, structural brain changes have been identified including hippocampal atrophy as well as frontal and caudate atrophy. Moreover, these structural brain changes have been associated with specific cognitive impairments.

Psychiatry's historical emphasis on psychotherapeutic approaches has been overtaken by what Michaels and Markowitz refer to as 'the remedicalization' of psychiatry. Treatment in psychiatry moved from a focus on providing 'therapy for the unhappiness and vicissitudes of life' towards a medically defined indication for treatment. The recent psychotherapeutic emphasis on short-term evidenced-based, manual-based therapies has also transformed the field of psychiatry and will also need to be adapted for an older population.

Age-based vs. needs-based services: the future of geriatrics?

There is no doubt that the behemoth of neuroscience cannot be ignored in the future development of old age psychiatry, particularly in terms of our understanding mental disorders and their treatment. However, clinical and service delivery issues will not be addressed adequately by the traditional approach of neurology or neuroscientists. For this, we must turn to the sister disciplines of geriatric psychiatry and geriatric medicine. In these sub specialties, recent debates, particularly in the UK, reflect the tension of developing age-based (geriatric) services versus disorder-based services that happen to be more prevalent in older adults. The recent Department of Health White Paper 'Securing better mental health for older adults' by Professors Ian Philp and Louis Appleby encapsulates this debate. The Department of Health attempted to provide a vision for the future of mainstream and specialist mental health services for older adults. This revealed a remarkably high prevalence of mental health difficulties in older adults which affect 40% of patients in general practice and half of general hospital patients. This high prevalence combined with the rapid growth of the elderly population, particularly the very old, make this an urgent public health matter. They note that 'age discrimination' in mental health services needs further attention so that services developed for working adults are available to older adults on the basis of need, not age. They note that one of the important functions of a specialist mental health service for older adults should include the support of colleagues in mainstream settings. Specialist services should also help to facilitate referral pathways to specialists and support services for older adults with mental illnesses. In this model, mental health and social care service provision for adults should be based on need and the right fit of intervention, rather than on age alone. They argue against an automatic transfer of patients from younger adult to older adult services simply because they pass the age of 65. Indeed, some younger adults who have multiple physical co-morbidities, cognitive impairment and frailty may be better served by older adult services. On the other hand, older adults who are otherwise physically fit and may have been known to adult services may best be served by the same adult service. However, older adults who present for the first time late in life with a major mental disorder are more likely to need old-age specialist services. The point of developing needs-based services is to ensure that service developments in one sector of the health care system do not have unintended adverse consequences for individuals who use the service in a different sector. In order for this to happen, government and local health services require a comprehensive vision for the health care service.

The position of the Department of Health advocating against age-based services brought a sharp response from the Faculty of Old Age Psychiatry in the UK. They counter that while the notion of age-inclusive services sounds equitable, they still fear that older adults will be excluded from these services for the same reasons that they were excluded before the development of POA. Moreover, the politically popular emphasis on 'choice' in future health services may not auger well for older adults. From the geriatric medical perspective, there is an added concern that 'choice' will further erode the capacity to recruit qualified geriatricians (see article by Metz and Labrooy, 2005 in the further reading section below). If older people are allowed to exercise choice, they may not see themselves as frail and may reject geriatric medical services in favour of mainstream adult services. They may indeed 'start voting with their feet'. This in turn would exacerbate a decline in demand for geriatric services and erode further an already weak academic base. There is a fear that by emphasizing 'choice' under the rubric of 'integration', older adults will only be given lip service in terms of access. Old-age psychiatrists and geriatric specialty services need to be advocates for older adults. Some have argued that to counter the impact of 'choice' and the erosion of the base of geriatrics, that geriatricians should take a lead in delivering hospital-based services that are of particular relevance to older people, including emphasis on conditions such as stroke, urinary incontinence and falls. Others have argued that geriatrics should be redefined as the clinical management of multiple long-term conditions. Indeed, the management of chronic disease is a priority in most developed health care services. Putting the emphasis on long-term chronic conditions may be easier to accept than simply being 'geriatric'.

Summary

Health services around the world face the challenge of a growing elderly population with a high prevalence of psychiatric and cognitive disorders. There is a growing consensus that clinical neurosciences must influence the future understanding and management of 'psychiatric' disorders in late life. However, the psychosocial perspective based in traditional psychiatry must be preserved both in terms of service delivery and instilling a holistic, humane and empathic approach to older adults, their families and caregivers. Diversity in approaches to this challenge will hopefully yield evidence-based and practical solutions that improve the quality of care of older individuals and families struggling to cope with these disorders. Determining whether the future of POA rests with the parent field of psychiatry, the newly developing field of clinical neurosciences, or the traditional field of 'geriatrics' remains a mug's game!

FURTHER READING

Articles

Cowan, W. M. and Kandel, E. R. (2001). Prospects for neurology and psychiatry. *JAMA*, **285**, 594–600.
Thoughtful article about the future of these two disciplines.

Insel, T. R. and Quirion, R. (2005). Psychiatry as a clinical neuroscience discipline. *JAMA*, **294**, 2221–2223.
These authors argue that psychiatry's future is as a neuroscience discipline.

Kandel, E. R. (1998). A new intellectual framework for psychiatry. *American Journal of Psychiatry*, **155**, 457–469.
See comments in text above.

Martin, J. (2002). The integration of neurology, psychiatry, and neuroscience in the 21st century. *American Journal of Psychiatry*, **159**, 695–704.
This article argues for the integration of these disciplines.

Mayberg, H. S. (2003). Modulating dysfunctional limbic–cortical circuits in depression: towards development of brain-based algorithms for diagnosis and optimized treatment. *British Medical Bulletin*, **65**, 193–207.
See text above.

Metz, D. H. and Labrooy, S. J. (2005). The future of geriatric medicine in an era of patient choice. *Age and Ageing*, **34**, 553–5535.
A frank discussion of the mess that geriatric medicine is in and possible ways out of the mire.

O'Brien, J. (2005). Dementia associated with psychiatric disorders. *International Psychogeriatrics,* **17** (Suppl. 1), S207–S221.
See text above.

Shulman, K. I. (1994). The future of geriatric psychiatry. *Canadian Journal of Psychiatry,* **39**, S4–8.
Earlier thoughts on this issue!

Index